Nursing Informatics

Guest Editor

JOY DON BAKER, PhD, RN-BC, CNE, CNOR, NEA-BC

PERIOPERATIVE NURSING CLINICS

www.periopnursing.theclinics.com

Consulting Editor
NANCY GIRARD, PhD, RN, FAAN

June 2012 • Volume 7 • Number 2

SAUNDERS an imprint of ELSEVIER, Inc.

W.B. SAUNDERS COMPANY
A Division of Elsevier Inc.

1600 John F. Kennedy Boulevard • Suite 1800 • Philadelphia, Pennsylvania 19103-2899

http://www.periopnursing.theclinics.com

PERIOPERATIVE NURSING CLINICS Volume 7, Number 2
June 2012 ISSN 1556-7931, ISBN-13: 978-1-4557-3914-1

Editor: Katie Hartner
Developmental Editor: Donald Mumford

Perioperative Nursing Clinics (ISSN 1556-7931) is published quarterly by Elsevier, 360 Park Avenue South, New York, NY 10010. Months of issue are March, June, September and December. Business and Editorial Offices: 1600 John F. Kennedy Blvd., Suite 1800, Philadelphia, PA 19103-2899. Customer Service Office: 11830 Westline Industrial Drive, St. Louis, MO 63146. Periodicals postage paid at New York, NY and at additional mailing offices. Subscription prices are $132.00 per year (domestic individuals), $224.00 per year (domestic institutions), $65.00.00 per year (domestic students/ residents), $171.00 per year (international individuals), $257.00 per year (international institutions), and $69.00 per year (International students/residents). Foreign air speed delivery is included in all *Clinics* subscription prices. All prices are subject to change without notice. **POSTMASTER:** Send change of address to *Perioperative Nursing Clinics,* Customer Service (orders, claims, online, change of address): Elsevier Periodicals Customer Service, 11830 Westline Industrial Drive, St. Louis, MO 63146. Tel: 1-800-654-2452 (U.S. and Canada). Fax: 314-523-5170. E-mail: journalscustomerservice-usa@elsevier.com (for print support); journalsonlinesupport-usa@elsevier.com (for online support).

Reprints. For copies of 100 or more, of articles in this publication, please contact the Commercial Rights Department, Elsevier Inc., 360 Park Avenue South, New York, NY 10010-1710; Phone: (+1) 212-633-3813; Fax: (+1) 212-462-1935; E-mail: reprints@elsevier.com.

Printed and bound by CPI Group (UK) Ltd, Croydon, CR0 4YY
Transferred to Digital Print 2012

Contributors

CONSULTING EDITOR

NANCY GIRARD, PhD, RN, FAAN
Nurse Collaborations, Boerne, Texas; Clinical Associate Professor, Acute Nursing Care Department, University of Texas Health Science Center, San Antonio, Texas

GUEST EDITOR

JOY DON BAKER, PhD, RN-BC, CNE, CNOR, NEA-BC
Clinical Associate Professor, Director, Distance Education; MSN/MPH Coordinator; College of Nursing, University of Texas at Arlington, Arlington, Texas

AUTHORS

JOY DON BAKER, PhD, RN-BC, CNE, CNOR, NEA-BC
Clinical Associate Professor, Director, Distance Education; MSN/MPH Coordinator; College of Nursing, University of Texas at Arlington, Arlington, Texas

KELLEY CONNOR, MS, RN
Assistant Professor, School of Nursing, Boise State University, Boise, Idaho

MICHELLE B. ECKHARD, RN, MSN
Chief Nursing Informatics Officer, Trinity Mother Frances Hospitals and Clinics, Tyler; Clinical Instructor, Graduate Nursing Administration Program, University of Texas at Arlington College of Nursing, Arlington, Texas

JOSHUA M. HAWKINS, BSN, RN, CPN
Clinical Health Record, Implementation and Optimization, Baylor Healthcare System, Dallas, Texas

HELEN HOUGH, MLS, BS, BA
Science and Nursing Librarian, Science and Engineering Library, University of Texas at Arlington, Arlington, Texas

DENISE JACKSON, MSN, RN, CNS-BC, CNOR, CRNFA
Clinical Nurse Specialist and Certified RN First Assistant, Shannon Clinic; Clinical Instructor, Post Graduate RNFA Program, Department of Nursing, Angelo State University, San Angelo, Texas

SARAH JONES, MA, MLS
Librarian, Digital Library Services, University of Texas at Arlington Library, Arlington, Texas

DELORES MARTIN, RN, CNOR, BSN
Operating Room Nurse, Surgical Services, Texas Health Allen Presbyterian Hospital, Allen, Texas

TONI MCKENNA, DNSc, RN
Director, Center for Continuing Nursing Education, University of Texas at Arlington, Arlington, Texas

PATRICIA NEWCOMB, RN, PhD, CPNP
Assistant Professor, College of Nursing; Director, Genomics Translational Research Lab, University of Texas at Arlington, Arlington, Texas

KRISTEN PRIDDY, RNC-OB, MSN, CNS
Clinical Instructor, College of Nursing, University of Texas at Arlington, Arlington, Texas

LANA RINGS, PhD
Associate Professor, College of Liberal Arts, Department of Modern Languages, University of Texas at Arlington, Arlington, Texas

EILEEN STEC, MS, MSW
Instruction and Outreach Librarian, Mabel Smith Douglass Library, Rutgers University, New Brunswick, New Jersey

NANCY ROPER WILLSON, RN, JD, MSN, MA
Attorney at Law, Assistant Clinical Professor, College of Nursing, University of Texas at Arlington, Arlington, Texas

Contents

> Nursing informatics is both a system and a science bringing order to all working elements. Health care has shifted from paper, to intranet, and today to Internet accessibility. The view of health care is changing to a synergistic and longitudinal focus on the perioperative patient including before and after a perioperative experience, but it is more a birth to death focus along with the lived health experiences in between. Nursing informatics is an integral part of the perioperative nursing practice.

> There is a renewed national focus on advancing the education levels of all nurses. Universities and colleges now offer online nursing courses and degree programs, which makes access to higher levels of education better than ever for perioperative nurses who want to return to school yet continue to work in the operating room. An understanding of the personal characteristics and technologic skills required for successful online learning will guide the decision-making process when considering the different delivery methods of nursing education.

> Technological changes affect patient care within the entire profession of nursing. The operative arena presents challenges for the perioperative nurses who must keep up with the technology, ensuring correct utilization of this technology to ensure quality patient care is delivered. The informatics nurse provides support to nurses and is called upon as a translator between nursing and the information technology department, while ensuring administrators have sufficient data to demonstrate the value of the technology required to safeguard the delivery of quality patient care.

> Health care providers do literature searches in order to find evidence-based answers to problems. No matter the question, the most efficient search retrieval process requires sequential analytic and linear thinking. A method of question analysis is provided so an efficient search can quickly yield quality materials. Some common tools and techniques used in literature searching are examined. Some research tools may be free online whereas others may require subscriptions. Located materials may also be available free online whereas others might have associated costs. Ways of accessing both free and more expensive tools and materials are discussed.

> The uneven quality of information available online can make assessing the information's value difficult. Websites are useful only when their content meets the needs of readers. The standards of relevancy and reliability applied in perioperative nursing research can also be applied to systematic website assessment. Relevancy is when the content meets the needs of viewers. Reliability can be assessed when there is information about the author and hosting site along with contact data, good spelling and grammar, and a creation date. Viewers have to trust their knowledge and determine if the information is accurate, objective, and supported by appropriate references.

> Busy perioperative nurses can manage nursing literature with the use of bibliographic management software, online databases and full-text journal articles. Two software products, EndNote and RefWorks, are compared for ease of use, cost, individual features and ability to search PubMed and Cumulative Index for Nursing and Allied Health Literature (CINAHL) databases.

> Every time a nurse gives a patient printed instructions to take home, makes photocopies to share with others, downloads a file or graphic to use at work, provides handouts at an in-service or a class, or writes for publication, issues related to copyright are involved. A basic understanding of why copyright exists, what it involves, and how it impacts the health care provider is important. Copyright fair use allows some flexibility. Failure to abide by copyright regulations can financially

impact both the provider and the institution where the provider works. Using this knowledge can protect the nurse from lawsuits.

Information management is a critical skill for professional nurses, but many staff nurses remain unaware of easily accessible tools for organizing and manipulating large amounts of data. This article briefly reviews the structures, purposes, and common applications of electronic spreadsheet and relational database programs that could be useful to practicing nurses. Examples are provided that reflect common situations encountered in perioperative nursing practice.

This article explores organizing categories as a framework for Personal Information Management (PIM). A brief exploration of the role of memory in PIM and rationale for using a predefined method for storage and retrieval of data are provided. Purposes for using a PIM system identified in this article are related to quality improvement, staff development, and patient and academic education. One application example assignment illustrates the use of file management to gather, store, and distribute evaluated Web sites. Barriers that must be overcome and benefits to PIM are also discussed.

This article describes the exciting adventure of planning and successfully implementing a continuing nursing education activity in a virtual world *(Second Life)* learning environment. The authors describe the challenges of providing continuing education and how experts can be brought together with learners in a virtual world. The authors discuss use of an orientation program to put learners at ease in the virtual world and understand navigation and avatar maneuvering. An outcome report shows the diversity of participants and their physical locations, as well as their constructive and positive feedback on the learning experience.

Perioperative nurses require ongoing education throughout their career to stay current in their practice. Although there are many formats available for nurses to gain continuing education knowledge, virtual reality may enhance current learning options. Virtual reality environments are flexible spaces in which users are able to interact with each other and the space around them. Virtual reality education options include both synchronous and asynchronous learning.

This article summarizes the challenges encountered when implementing an electronic health record (EHR) in a perioperative setting. Barriers and facilitators and generational differences are discussed. Strategies for mitigation of these barriers are discussed using specific examples. In addition, real-world perspectives from perioperative nurses who have been heavily involved in implementation are offered.

With platforms such as *Second Life,* simulation training in virtual environments is possible within distance learning. Yet, along with opportunities come challenges, both technological and intercultural, to providing access to such learning. This article discusses technological and intercultural opportunities and challenges related to simulation learning in virtual environments for perioperative nursing education. It describes current thinking regarding the needs, beneficial uses, and caveats for virtual simulation learning. It also addresses the importance of culturally appropriate nonverbal and verbal communicative behavior within the contexts of learning, virtual environments, and professional practice.

Nurses owe a duty to their patients to provide safe nursing care. Posting information concerning patient incidents, whether such posting rises to the level of being considered a Health Insurance Portability and Accountability Act of 1996 violation, is frequently viewed as a failure to maintain the professional boundary. A common element is that the nurse is fatigued, stressed, and overwhelmed and unwisely uses the social networking site to vent frustration. There are a number of helpful resources to assist nurses in gaining greater understanding of this topic, including the guide published by the National Council of State Boards of Nursing.

PERIOPERATIVE NURSING CLINICS

Preface

Nursing Informatics

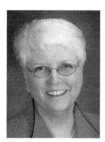

Joy Don Baker, PhD, RN-BC, CNE, CNOR, NEA-BC
Guest Editor

Technology fills the everyday life of the perioperative registered nurse (RN) and informatics is an integral reality of our practice. Teaching Informatics in the university provides a rich opportunity of diverse encounters between practicing nursing professionals seeking education and those seeking to facilitate learning. Therefore, the opportunity to use ideas from my own practice began to surface when first asked to serve in the role of guest editor for this *Perioperative Nursing Clinics* issue. The recent Institute of Medicine (IOM) report[1] emphasis on information systems to support nursing practice is an element critical to this issue and my own practice.

Another key element of the IOM report is the advancement of nurses and the continual academic progression of the lifelong learner.[1] Perioperative RNs holding associate degrees are returning to school and using online means to access the education paths. As nurses return to school, they face a myriad of options. This *Perioperative Nursing Clinics* issue addresses the question "what is nursing informatics?" and its applicability to nursing practice. The narrative also addresses the distinction between the synchronous and asynchronous styles of online education. As new roles emerge, a relationship develops with the individuals in practice, education, and administration to accomplish the outcomes desired.

Another question develops around the need and desire to make perioperative practice decisions based on the most current and relevant literature. Delving into the literature can be exciting and exasperating, and tips for improving strategies as well as the means by which they are evaluated can be found in this issue. In addition, this issue addresses the options of how and where bibliographic information might be stored so that it is accessible for use in both the immediate present and future. Ease of accessing information also plays into the issues of implementation of an electronic health record and is no longer a luxury of the few; it is a requirement and the processes are critical to the perioperative patient, nurse, and the future expectations of one's personal health record.

As a result and for ease of access to materials, images, and so forth, perioperative nurses wish to share materials among each other and with their patients. The

Perioperative Nursing Clinics 7 (2012) xi–xii
doi:10.1016/j.cpen.2012.03.002
1556-7931/12/$ – see front matter **periopnursing.theclinics.com**

dissemination of information is a constant critical need for perioperative RNs; however, to accomplish this without encroaching on the authors' or developers' rights is a concern that surfaces and is addressed in the issue. There is also a variety of data management ideas provided within the various articles.

Opportunities for using virtual reality environments for continuing education and simulation purposes are explored in both the academic and the practice settings. Concepts surrounding social networking and the cultural issues of living in a cyberworld are found in the pages of this issue. Do we as perioperative nurses clearly understand the ramifications of social networking? The perception of boundaries is a concept often taught in nursing school, particularly as it relates to the patient. As perioperative nurses, we also have to clearly understand and interpret the boundaries of professional and personal social networking and the effects this has on one's career.

The wonderful contributors to this *Perioperative Nursing Clinics* issue on Nursing Informatics developed rich and in-depth concepts. They represent a diversity of practices and professions from across the United States. Their expertise and willingness to share their knowledge provided solid strength, making the culmination of their collective work a powerful contribution for those of us within perioperative nursing. For the insightful work they have done, I am deeply indebted and offer my heartfelt thanks.

Joy Don Baker, PhD, RN-BC, CNE, CNOR, NEA-BC
College of Nursing
University of Texas at Arlington
Box 19407
411 South Nedderman Drive
Arlington, TX 76019-0407, USA

E-mail address:
jdbaker@uta.edu

REFERENCE

1. Institute of Medicine [IOM]. The future of nursing: Leading change, advancing health. Washington, DC: The National Academies of Press; 2011.

Nursing Informatics

Joy Don Baker, PhD, RN-BC, CNE, CNOR, NEA-BC

KEYWORDS

- Informatics • Accessibility • Information system • Computer system • Nursing science
- Cognitive science

KEY POINTS

- Nursing informatics is both a system and a science.
- Shift in health care system from experiential to longitudinal focus.
- Application opportunities for informatics in perioperative practice, administration, education, and research.
- Issues of accessibility represent both challenges and opportunities.

Nursing informatics (NI) is both a system and a science. A system brings order or method and is a coordinated arrangement of working elements or organisms.[1,2] Science is a systematic acquisition of knowledge, especially knowledge that can be precisely measured. If we think of body systems such as cardiovascular, respiratory, skin, and so forth, none of these can operate independent of the other, and often controlling or supporting changes in related systems. NI functions in the same way. A system may also use science to acquire knowledge for precise measurement just as the body uses incremental changes in blood flow, which will change the extremity vascular system outcome. NI uses both a system process and scientific data.

SELECTED NURSING INFORMATICS DEFINITIONS

In 1994, the American Nurses Association (ANA) began developing a statement to describe the scope of practice for NI: "The development and evaluation of applications, tools, processes, and structures which assist nurses with the management of data in taking care of patients or supporting the practice of nursing."[3,4] This foundational work supported the need and importance of NI related to the practice of nursing. Then in 1996, Turley[5] framed NI, identifying the sciences reflected in NI. The overlapping concepts of the Venn diagram (**Fig. 1**) demonstrate the center where NI is represented.

In 1998, the Nursing Informatics Special Interest Group of International Medical Informatics Association[6] also developed a definition: "The integration of nursing, its

The author has nothing to disclose.

College of Nursing, University of Texas at Arlington, Box 19407, 411 South Nedderman Drive, Arlington, TX 76019-0407, USA

E-mail address: jdbaker@uta.edu

Perioperative Nursing Clinics 7 (2012) 151–160
doi:10.1016/j.cpen.2012.02.010
1556-7931/12/$ – see front matter © 2012 Elsevier Inc. All rights reserved.

periopnursing.theclinics.com

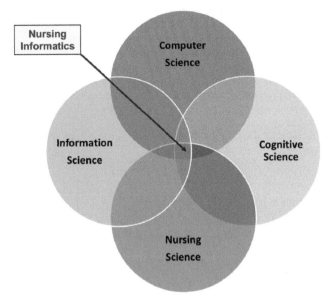

Fig. 1. Nursing informatics Venn diagram. (*Adapted from* Turley JP. Toward a model of nursing informatics. Image J Nurs Sch 1996;28[1]:6.)

information, and information management with information processing and communication technology, to support the health of people worldwide."[6] Then in 2001 (**Box 1**), ANA developed a more detailed definition focusing on the three science legs of NI; nursing science, computer science, and information science. NI is the facilitator of the integration of data that supports our patients related to nursing decision-making. We do that in everyday work; therefore, the definition of NI is being built on what we do in nursing practice. The structures, the processes, and the added information technology make up the foundational pieces that support what NI is to nursing practice.[7,4]

In 2008, ANA[8] enhanced iterations of the NI definition.

"Nursing informatics (NI) is the specialty that integrates nursing science, computer science, and information science to manage and communicate data, information, knowledge, and wisdom in nursing practice. Nursing informatics

---

Box 1
ANA 2001 definition of nursing informatics

"A specialty that integrates *nursing science*, *computer science*, and *information science* to manage and communicate data, information, and knowledge in nursing practice.

Nursing informatics facilitates the *integration of data*, information and knowledge to *support patients*, nurses and other providers in their *decision-making* in all roles and settings.

This support is accomplished through the use of information *structures*, information *processes*, and information *technology*."

From American Nurses Association. Scope and standards of nursing informatics practice. Washington, DC: American Nurses Association; 2001.

facilitates the integration of data, information, knowledge, and wisdom to support patients, nurses, and other providers in their decision-making in all roles and settings. This support is accomplished through the use of information structures, information processes, and information technology."[8]

We collect data or facts that may be reported without interpretation such as blood pressure, pulse rate, temperatures, and so forth, but if nothing is done with the data or there is no interpretation of what they mean, then data become of little value. Computer science deals with the organization of the data by collecting, storing, processing, retrieving, and displaying information as well as communicating the information.[9] This process is done with hardware, software, various platforms, portals for data collection and retrieval, and components necessary for the computer science portion of NI.

Information science is the processing systems associated with placing data into relative and meaningful statements.[10] The data cannot stand by itself, it must have the information processed and then analyzed within the information system science. From there the knowledge through cognitive science allows involvement demonstrating developing interrelationships among informational statements to create a meaningful whole yielding cognition and knowledge or perception. Informatics combines computer and informational science in order to manage and process data, information, and knowledge that then lead to actions by the perioperative nurse.

THEORIES SUPPORTING NURSING INFORMATICS

Burns and Grove[11] describe theory as consisting "of an integrated set of defined concepts, existence statements, and relational statements that present a view of phenomenon and can be used to describe, explain, predict, or control that phenomenon."[11] There are theories that inform and help frame NI such as general systems theory and cybernetics, cognitive theory, and change theory.

Systems or general systems theory[1] has been discussed earlier in this article and has to do with interacting parts within some form of a boundary.[1] Boundaries are present all the time and are dealt with routinely. The body itself is a boundary for housing our body parts and organs. Each of the parts of a human, bounded by the skin and utilizing the skeletal frame, all come together to make a whole. Cybernetics (controlled system)[1,12] theory is "based on communication (transfer of information) between system and environment and within the system, and control (feedback) of the system's function in regard to environment."[1] That process might be similar to that of a thermostat in our home where there is an opportunity to set high and low parameters for the system to adjust automatically to keep it in the preset range. Perioperative nurses use cardiac monitors that allow high/low parameters to be established to cause alarms to signal a problem is at hand for the nurse to take action.

Information and communications are areas that relate to how the computer groups data, information, and knowledge input into the system. There is a connection to these elements of storage relative to cognitive theory as it incorporates information input, processing, and output relative to short- and long-term learning, memory, and skills. Change theory also comes into direct play as health care facilities increase their use of electronic health records (EHR). Lewin's[13] force field theory is a sequence of unfreezing from the current situation, moving toward the new reality, and finally refreezing so the new change is a part of practice and no longer seen as new. For example, the perioperative setting where the perioperative patient record is being migrated from an all-paper system to an electronic format can represent a fairly static or frozen state of being for nurses steeped in the paper tradition. The change occurs,

---

Box 2
Selected nursing and health care data elements and sets

Standard Terminology Acceptable in Electronic Health Record

Perioperative Nursing Data Set (PNDS)
Patient Care Data Set (PCDS)
Home Health Care Classification (HHCC)
Omaha System
North American Nursing Diagnostic Association (NANDA)
Nursing Intervention Classification (NIC)
Nursing Outcomes Classification (NOC)
Nursing Management Minimum Data Set (NMMDS)
Systematized Nomenclature of Medicine - Reference Terminology (SNOMED RT)

---

and after a time the new EHR is established into the setting, and the nurse has learned and solidified (refrozen) the method into his/her practice.

HEALTH CARE SYSTEM SHIFT

Health care has been transitioning for several years now, from a traditional system or somewhat of a stand-alone system into a more information-driven system. Constantly we are asked for data to support opinions or ideas. Information is the foundation on which we make our decisions. Therefore, information is critical to the outcome, and the method used involves both the computer systems and information systems. The information management of those systems becomes imperative. Nurses think about patients from a whole-being mindset from birth to death, or a longitudinal process. However, in hospitals in the past we tended to think of one patient experience, that moment in time; we chart everything related to that situation, and then we may never see the patient again. In a longitudinal process, we are looking for how this experience relates to the whole patient over his/her whole life. These mindsets represent the variations from our past to a much more current theme and approach to health care from traditional to information-driven systems.

NURSING ROLE

In 2009, 60% of all nurses worked within the hospital setting.[14] Perioperative registered nurses (RNs) work in interdependent practice environments relying heavily on information access, data transfer, innovative patient interaction, and communication systems for accountable and measurable care outcomes. Perioperative nurses work with their health professional colleagues in informatics, information systems, and computer technology to create systems that are capable of storing, collecting, and analyzing the data into meaningful elements for the nurses' use. The analysis reports from the collected data are then evaluated for opportunities to improve on the practice processes and systems, allowing the nurse to better meet patient needs.

NURSING DATA ELEMENTS AND SETS

Terms are defined so that single-structured data elements are used within the charting process. This strategy allows for the care that is provided patients to be documented and provides a quality way for the care to be effectively evaluated. **Box 2** represents a sample list of languages that are currently in use by nurses, such as

Nursing Intervention Classification (NIC), Nursing Outcomes Classification (NOC), and North American Nursing Diagnostic Association (NANDA). Perhaps less familiar are the specialty organizations' data elements and nomenclature development involved in the process over time, such as that of the Perioperative Nursing Data Set (PNDS).

The PNDS is a nomenclature germane to the practice of perioperative nursing. Creating a nomenclature is a lengthy process, and specialty organizations such as the Association of periOperative Registered Nurses (AORN, Inc.) do not want to *reinvent the wheel,* but rather to build on what is already established and at the same time explore what is germane to the specialty. That language then needs to be a part of the total system so all perioperative nurses are using the same definitions in the same way for the same function, item, or activity. It is therefore critical for these types of elements to be developed to provide the basis for effectiveness related to evaluation of outcomes. For example, using consistent language for procedure start time and exit time provides a method to compare data results across hospital systems for quality improvement.

NURSING APPLICATIONS
Practice

Nursing information systems can be applied to nursing practice in ways such as work lists, client documentation, monitoring devices, care plan and critical pathways, automatic billing with nursing documentation, reminders during documentation to aid charting, and quick accessibility regarding patient data from previous encounters. This is not an exclusive list, it is simply offered as an example of the ways nursing practice implements the use of information systems. Consider this perioperative scenario: a patient arrives in the patient holding area prior to surgery short of breath and complaining of chest pain. Describe how informatics can help the perioperative RN and other health care providers more efficiently and effectively care for this patient. Whether taking a very broad approach in the conceptual thinking or very specific, the issue is to think through what is being used from an information systems standpoint. Consider things such as the old patient records, including medical history, and medications that are available at the touch of a fingertip today. High quality care is readily available through telemedicine, electronically submitted electrocardiograms, chest radiographs, and on-call specialists that might be off-site. Perhaps the latest research on the patient's drugs and presenting symptoms are available via the Internet. Expert systems and care maps guide the treatment plan. These are methods for using various information systems in perioperative practice.

Administration

Information systems are constantly being used in nursing administration. I know of few managers who do not rely heavily on staffing scheduling systems. E-mail is a feature almost all of us use to aid communications via our phone system and laptops. The cost and trending analysis for budgeting purposes is imperative to have solid data to make decisions, and data are what drives the whole process. If improvements are to be made to quality services provided, then looking for the desired outcomes data to support our opinions is imperative. Administrators' use of data helps reinforce the opinions on what is happening around them to determine the path and direction of change they are choosing for system improvements.

Education

Nursing education is using information systems routinely, from face-to-face simulation to online simulation opportunities. The Internet is the lifeline to other countries and identifying the best possible ways and means to access data not available in the past to accomplish the desired outcomes. Computerized record-keeping, computer-assisted instruction, distance learning via teleconferencing, Internet resources, and Web-based education, along with presentation software all support the continued advancement of nursing education.

Experiential learning concepts are about concrete experience, observation, and reflection, in which generalizations are formulated about situations and patients that have lasting implications for nursing practice. In addition, any new situation encountered influences this generalization. Reflection then is a conceptual tool for understanding variation, differences, and ambiguity, and then putting them all into a framework that makes them understandable. Reflection **IN** action is, for example, the reflection occurring when providing care to a patient. A reflection **IN** action might be when a student nurse is giving an injection for the first time. How does it make students feel; are they nervous or calm, is it working for them to be able to give the injection, or is panic taking over? A new employee in the perioperative setting in a new situation is performing a new activity; what is his/her first reaction in that moment of time? It is his/her own self-reflection of the experience as it is occurring that is a reflection **IN** action of that particular moment in time?

Reflection **ON** action is taking place after the learning or event has occurred. For example, during the post conference of a group of students or new nurses the instructor asks them to interpret their practice for that day related to information systems. What did they use, how did they use it, and why did they use information systems to accomplish their responsibilities and tasks? Their responses would be a reflection **ON** action.

Reflection **FOR** action is where the individual is reflecting on what opportunities exist for change and improvement in the future. *How will I incorporate those changes for improvement into my future practice? Based on what was learned from the experience, what action will be taken for improvement?* Those three elements: reflection **IN, ON**, and **FOR** action, are the makeup of an experiential learning activity.[15]

There are five *E*s of electronic education, and those are experiential learning, engagement, empowerment, electronics, and evaluation. *Engagement* is the understanding of the process of learning, which means there is engagement by the student, and it is crucial for learning to happen. The learner must be able to influence what is being learned. There must be active and engaged learning taking place for knowledge to be gained. *Empowerment* means distribution of responsibility among all participants including students, teachers, and the educational activity. The faculty/staff development instructor needs to be the *guide on the side* versus the person who is performing all of the content delivery and serving as a *sage on stage*. The learner needs to be able to share that responsibility with the teacher for the process of learning to take place. *Electronic*, use of information technology in educational activities such as the use of Second Life or ConnectPro, provide Internet-based simulation and communication opportunity. *Evaluation* and the reflection on processes and outcomes are critical components of electronic education. Similar and related to what is happening in an "in the seat" environment, it is imperative that the evaluation occur in the electronic environment as well.

Reflection on process evaluation related to education fits in both the hospital and the academic settings. Individuals who are being asked to share their thoughts on evaluation of the process are students in academic settings and patients within the hospital setting. What is the satisfaction level and were the outcomes expected actually achieved by the participant in this case? Process evaluation also includes the faculty/nurse and the facility such as the hospital, clinic, or classroom. How did the process meet or not meet the needs of the specific individual? The reflection on outcomes has to do with whether the action taken accomplished the original target or established benchmark. Measurements of cost means did the cost outweigh the benefits, and if that is the case, then how to go about adjusting the process to help change the outcome result. Monitoring the number of participants enrolled or participating in the continuing education event addresses one area related to determining a return on investment for conducting the classes.

This reflective evaluation process occurs in the perioperative setting, for example, the numbers of first case start times over the previous year may be an example of meeting a targeted outcome. Were data provided to surgeons that had an impact on their behavior for arriving in the operating room on time, resulting in an increase in on-time case starts? Infection rates, mortality, and morbidity are other indicators that are used to establish reflection on outcomes. The desired outcomes or benchmark are determined first, the activities are completed, and the evaluation occurs in relation to the preset targets.

Research

Nursing research is another application for information systems. An interesting side note, CINAHL (Cumulative Index to Nursing and Allied Literature) in 1940 started out as a series of index cards, and not until 1984 did it move into an online database.[16] The means for searching the literature was finding the index card, then finding the hard copy article in the library stacks in order to be able to find relevant materials. That process has gone from the index cards that would lead the perioperative nurse to the journal stacks to now having the full-text journal articles accessible to nurses via the Internet. The transition has been phenomenal. The adoption of standardized languages related to nursing terms has been able to help drill down into the searching process in order to find significant articles that meet the needs of the topic being researched. The ability to find trends and aggregated data also allows us to look at large populations of groups using a variety of different databases such as computerized literature searching using CINAHL, CHIN (Community Health Information Networks) or MEDLINE/PubMed ("MEDLINE® contains journal citations and abstracts for biomedical literature from around the world. PubMed® provides free access to MEDLINE and links to full text articles when possible"[17]). The Internet has become a way of obtaining, collecting, and conducting research. It provides the means to ask the questions about perioperative practice such as how to change the practice or if the current practice is the best practice possible for the patients.

ROADBLOCKS AND CHALLENGES VERSUS OPPORTUNITIES AND TRENDS

There are multiple roadblocks and challenges faced when new opportunities and trends begin to demonstrate themselves relative to NI. However, with information systems, one of the things to consider is how to change these challenges and roadblocks into opportunities for new and innovative ideas. Access is a part of this issue such as *freedom of use* versus *security of information*. We must work with the Health Insurance and Portability Act guidelines and for universities the Family Education Rights and Privacy Act guidelines. The main question is who has the right to use the items or information and who does not. Giving access to the individuals who need it without breaching the confidentiality of patients and restricting others from accessing who should not have the information is a key debatable item. One current negative trend is the issue of lack of privacy or feeling like *big brother* is watching and accessing one's personal information without the person's knowledge or consent. In our environment of threats to our society and our personal information and identity managing, these types of issues are affecting our practice and our society.

Something never experienced ultimately becomes an opportunity, even though initially it may be approached with a degree of trepidation. For example, a person exiting an elevator in the hospital observes a robot, Pyxis, moving down the hall unassisted. The Pyxis stopped if it encountered people or made adjustments if the hallway shifted, and it moved on down the hall until it came to the nurses' station where it stopped and waited for a nurse to receive the unit. A fascinating process to observe for the first time as well as to see potential reduction in transport and pharmacy delivery labor costs. A balancing of how does the system work, does the technology meet the need, is it secure, and is it a change that is beneficial to everyone involved are questions that must be addressed when implementing innovative technology. Determining whether it is the right thing to do for the right reasons and for the people involved are essential questions to determine and evaluate the outcome of the new technology.

Define Information Accessibility

Information accessibility means information is available regardless of the platform or the user agent. As the population moves away from the personal computer to other user agents such as the smart phone, iPad, and personal digital assistant for communications, information accessibility should increase. Electronic books represent another form of user agent that assists individuals in accessing information. Strict adherence to design guidelines is required by the developers, such as using consistent language when writing the programs and following established standards.

Rendition means the presentation method on the screen, such as does the information show up as a cascading format, does it open into a new window, and how does it appear on the screen for the user. Disability is again a key component, and there are five elements that must be addressed in order to meet all American with Disability Act (ADA) issues. Those aspects are visual, hearing, mobility, cognitive or knowledge, and seizure.[18] Information accessibility relates specifically to the user and then moves into the platform and user agent. The computer technology and information systems developments advance society to make information accessible for everyday use.

Accessibility Change Issues

Have you ever used a wheelchair ramp to go into a building because it was simply easier than going up the stairs, particularly if you are carrying a large load or pulling luggage? Have you used an elevator instead of stairs or listened to audio tapes instead of reading the book? These innovations developed for physical, appliance, or accessibility issues are based on disabilities and may ultimately be used by people other than those with the originating issue that it was created. Accessibility is often more than the originating disability phenomenon and generates discussions such as those regarding access to buildings. In 1973, the Rehabilitation Act[18,19] was implemented, and at that time injured veterans were returning from the Vietnam War. We were in a process where we needed to do things differently than in the past. The process used in the past no longer met the physical needs, and something had to be done.

Appliances are items used to support people but may/may not be used from a physical standpoint. That appliance might be something like a screen reader for the blind. Audio tapes of both music and books are another form of appliance used to support individuals with sight impairment. However, consider how often they are used on a daily bases by drivers particularly on long trips, offsetting the radio or in areas where the radio is not accessible. This practice keeps the driver and his/her hands on the steering wheel, allows a little entertainment, and at that same time the driver can focus on the road. The disability of limited sight or no vision may have generated the need in the first place; however, appliances of this nature often become used by the general population as well.

In the early 1990s, information access was becoming less of an issue on an internal basis because of the widespread use of computers. Those systems have been changing, and now the Internet is used for a more diverse and wider based option than in those years. It is important to understand that these innovations were coming out of a need to help people access buildings, utilize appliances that provided mobility, and access to information. The innovations were driven initially by disability but are now used routinely by the greater population.

Importance of Accessibility

Information accessibility success is important to higher education, administrators, patients, and clinical practice. Think about the shift of education materials from paper-based to Web-based. Fewer organizations are copying materials for hard-copy delivery; it is being done via electronic distribution. The use of nonpersonal computer user agents such as smart phones and iPads is increasing. In order to stay apprised of the changing information flow, one must have access.

The last area is the law that mandates accessibility. However, the law is not the best reason to make changes; it is better to do it simply because it is the right thing to do. If we think about who benefits from making information accessible, the law was originally intended for individuals with some form of impairment, but it provides us opportunities for separate content from a different rendition, which may make it easier for anyone to understand the information differently and with more clarity. The process provides a predictable set of rules for adaptive technology access, meaning that the access must meet all of the ADA criteria. In 1990, ramps were mandated in new construction.[18] Compliance occurred because of the law **and** it was the right thing to do. This change made access to buildings easier and safer for people. Universal design can increase access for all, not just those with a particular disability. Information accessibility becomes a critical component that perioperative nurses must address with each new encounter.

SUMMARY

Give thought to how informatics are applied in perioperative practice; how we teach, organize work groups, and communicate information to patients. The everyday practice is integrated with NI to allow us to improve patient outcomes by reviewing data, evaluation strategies, and testing working assumptions and theories. Perioperative RNs use computer technology when posting patient assessments to the EHR. They incorporate information science as they gather trend data to make knowledgeable (cognitive) decisions well-supported from the nursing science literature (see **Fig. 1**). We do not always give conscious thought to the NI supporting us behind the scenes, unless it is not working, any more than we consciously think about the stethoscope we use to listen to a patient's lungs or heart. However, without these supporting tools and systems we would be quite lost. It is the balance of technology, knowledge, and the art of nursing that makes up quality outcomes for patients.

REFERENCES

1. Bertalanffy LV. General system theory: foundations, development, applications. New York: George Braziller; 1968.

2. Kitson AL. The need for systems change: reflections on knowledge translation and organizational change. J Adv Nurs 2008;65(1):217–28.
3. American Nurses Association. The scope of practice for nursing informatics [ANA publication NP-907.5M 5/94]. Washington, DC: American Nurses Association; 1994.
4. Staggers N, Thompson CB. The evolution of definitions for nursing informatics: a critical analysis and revised definition. J Am Med Inform Assoc 2002;9(3):255–61.
5. Turley JP. Toward a model of nursing informatics. Image J Nurs Sch 1996;28(1):309–13.
6. Special Interest Group of International Medical Informatics Association Nursing Informatics (IMIA-NI). IMIA-NI General Assembly 1998 Minutes. Proceedings of the General Assembly Meeting. Seoul, Korea, August 19, 1998.
7. American Nurses Association. Scope and standards of nursing informatics practice. Washington, DC: American Nurses Association; 2001.
8. American Nurses Association. Nursing Informatics: scope and standards of practice. Silver Spring (MD): American Nurses Association; 2008. p. i–216.
9. Department of Computer Science. What is computer science? Published 2003. Available at: http://www.cs.bu.edu/AboutCS/WhatIsCS.pdf. Accessed January 14, 2012.
10. Department of Engineering. Information Science and Engineering Department. Published 2010. Available at: http://www.seaedu.ac.in/insciengg.html. Accessed January 14, 2012,
11. Burns N, Grove SK. The practice of nursing research: conduct, critique, and utilization. 5th edition. St Louis (MO): Elsevier Saunders; 2005. p. 37.
12. University of Reading: School of Engineering. What is cybernetics? Available at: http://www.reading.ac.uk/sse/about/cyber/cyber-whatiscybernetics.aspx. Accessed January 24, 2012.
13. Lewin K. Field Theory in Social Science. New York: Harper & Row; 1951.
14. Bureau of Labor Statistics, US Department of Labor. Occupational outlook handbook, 2010-11 edition, registered nurses. Available at: http://www.bls.gov/oco/ocos083.htm. Accessed January 24, 2012.
15. Knowles M, Holton E, Swanson RA. The adult learner. 5th edition. Woburn (MA): Butterworth-Heinemann; 1998.
16. Lincoln Memorial University Library. N430 nursing research: CINAHL history then and now. Published 2006. Available at: http://www.google.com/url?sa=t&rct=j&q=cinahl%20history&source=web&cd=1&ved=0CB4QFjAA&url=http%3A%2F%2Flibrary.lmunet.edu%2Fwp-content%2Fuploads%2F2009%2F01%2Fcinahl-history.doc&ei=JkofT-vID6GQ2QXQ24WxDw&usg=AFQjCNHH28oPCxrKLjb8tgrtmWKuv9hAcA. Accessed January 24, 2012.
17. US National Library of Medicine, National Institutes of Health. Medline/PubMed. Available at: http://www.nlm.nih.gov/bsd/pmresources.html. Accessed January 24, 2012.
18. Department of Justice. Americans With Disabilities Act of 1990, as amended. Published 2009. Available at: http://www.ada.gov/pubs/ada.htm. Accessed January 24, 2012.
19. US Department of Justice, Civil Rights Division, and Disability Rights Section. A guide to disability rights laws: Rehabilitation Act. Published 2005. Available at: http://www.ada.gov/cguide.htm#anchor65610. Accessed January 24, 2012.

Synchronous Versus Asynchronous Online Courses:
An Introduction for Perioperative Nurses Returning to School

Denise Jackson, MSN, RN, CNS-BC, CNOR, CRNFA[a,b,*]

KEYWORDS

- Online nursing education • Synchronous • Asynchronous • Perioperative

KEY POINTS

- Obtaining a BSN or MSN has become an important factor in advancement for perioperative nurses.
- Nursing schools are helping to provide access to higher education by offering an online format.

In October 2010, the Institute of Medicine released its landmark report—*The Future of Nursing: Leading Change, Advancing Health.*[1] As a result of this report, the profession of nursing has come together in an unprecedented and collaborative effort to move the recommendations made in the report forward. The 4 key messages of the report are:

- Nurses should practice to the full extent of their education and training
- Nurses should achieve higher levels of education and training through an improved education system that promotes seamless academic progression
- Nurses should be full partners, with physicians and other health professionals, in redesigning health care in the United States
- Effective workforce planning and policy making require better data collection and an improved information infrastructure.[1]

The 8 recommendations of the report are:

- Remove scope-of-practice barriers
- Expand opportunities for nurses to lead and diffuse collaborative improvement efforts

The author has nothing to disclose.
[a] Shannon Clinic, 120 East Beauregard, San Angelo, TX 76903, USA
[b] Department of Nursing, Angelo State University, 333 Vanderventer Avenue, San Angelo, TX 76909, USA
* Shannon Clinic, 120 East Beauregard, San Angelo, TX 76903.
E-mail address: kjackson2@angelo.edu

Perioperative Nursing Clinics 7 (2012) 161–169
doi:10.1016/j.cpen.2012.02.001   periopnursing.theclinics.com
1556-7931/12/$ – see front matter © 2012 Elsevier Inc. All rights reserved.

- Implement nurse residency programs
- Increase the proportion of nurses with a baccalaureate degree to 80% by 2020
- Double the number of nurses with a doctorate by 2020
- Ensure that nurses engage in lifelong learning
- Prepare and enable nurses to lead change to advance health
- Build an infrastructure for the collection of analysis of interprofessional health care workforce data.[1]

With regulatory agencies' intensified focus on quality, safety, access to care, and cost containment, it is more important than ever to ensure that the perioperative nurses of tomorrow are equipped with the knowledge and skills necessary to positively affect patient outcomes. It is also important that the perioperative nurses of today remain competent, are lifelong learners, and are equipped to be nursing leaders by obtaining higher levels of education. Health care reform and the Institute of Medicine report have generated a renewed focus on nursing education. This focus has resulted in a concentrated effort by nursing educators to find ways to facilitate seamless progression from 1 academic level to the next for all nurses.

The interest in obtaining a bachelor's or master's degree has never been greater for perioperative nurses. However, having an interest is often the stopping point for many nurses who want to advance their education, because they are unable and possibly even unwilling to leave the operating room setting to pursue their education goals. Demanding work schedules that offer little flexibility, financial constraints, family obligations, and an individual's physical location (with no proximity to a university) are all potential barriers for perioperative nurses.[2] Schools of nursing are providing much-needed access to higher education by developing new curriculum or by converting their current programs and delivering in an online format.[2,3] With this shift to online course delivery, perioperative nurses have been given a key to open doors that will take them to higher levels of education without taking them out of the operating room.

For the experienced nurse looking to return to school, the terms used to describe technology and delivery methods of curriculum can seem almost like a foreign language. The task of deciding which type of distance education program in which to enroll can be arduous. Selecting a program that best fits the busy schedule of perioperative nurses can be easier when there is an understanding of common terminology and options for course delivery.

DISTANCE EDUCATION

Distance education has been defined as any learning environment in which the student or learner is in a different location than the instructor.[4] There are different methods of course delivery under the broadly defined term *distance education*. Examples of early distance education are correspondence courses and independent, self-directed study projects. In correspondence courses, the exchange of educational materials, such as the course syllabus with guidelines for meeting specific academic objectives, completed student assignments, and instructor feedback, occurs via postal service, fax, email, or telephone. Examinations are administered to the student by a proctor located near the student's home. Correspondence courses are self-paced, and may or may not be tied to academic semesters with specific deadlines for completion.[4] Independent, self-directed study projects are negotiated and arranged between a student and a faculty member. The student selects the topic to study and formulates learning objectives. Together, the student and faculty identify learning resources, determine how the objectives will be met, and agree on how learning will be evaluated. This information, as well as how much credit will be awarded for successful completion of the study, are put in a learning contract signed by the student and faculty.[5]

Some courses utilize technology to enhance the learning experience by putting course materials online for students to access, but they still have a traditional *face-to-face* component in which the student and instructor are physically present in the same location. These courses are referred to as *blended* or *hybrid* classes.[4] Over the last decade, major advances in technology and communications have provided universities and colleges with the capability to transform traditional *face-to-face* academic courses, and even entire degree programs, into offerings that are Web based, delivered online, and take place in a virtual classroom.

Online course delivery is often divided into 2 distinct methods: asynchronous and synchronous. Understanding the differences between these 2 delivery methods is an important first step in selecting how to proceed with advancing one's educational goals. Each method has its own benefits and challenges and uses different techniques for students and faculty to communicate and interact. Each method requires different technologic skills for both the instructor and the student.

Synchronous Online Courses

Synchronous online courses are Web based. They are similar to traditional *face-to-face* course delivery methods because the teacher and the learner are in the same virtual classroom at the same time. Physical presence is not required, but virtual presence is. Common methods utilized to be *present* in class are Webinars, audio/video conferencing with and without whiteboards, chat rooms, and instant messaging.

Webinars

Webinars are presented in real time and use a combination of telephone conferencing for listening to the presenter and an Internet connection for viewing the presentation. Many newer computers come from the factory equipped with Voice over Internet Protocol (VoIP) and the capability to stream the audio portion over the Internet allowing the user to hear the lecture on their computer rather than dialing in to the conference via telephone.[6] Webinars can be interactive. They may also be unidirectional, in other words, the lecturer presents and the participants listen.

In large groups, presenters may select the option to mute the microphones or phone lines of the students while they are presenting. This is helpful to ensure that outside noises from the attendees' phone lines do not distract other students from listening to the presentation. If the groups are smaller, 2-way audio may be left open so listeners can ask questions.

Another way to communicate during Webinars is through instant messaging. Attendees can type their comments/questions in a designated chat box and then send them to the presenter's computer screen. The presenter has the option to address the questions privately through instant messaging or, ideally, will read the question out loud and provide an answer so the entire class can benefit from receiving the information.

Video conferencing

Video conferencing occurs in real time and is therefore used in synchronous online class delivery. Live, *face-to-face* interaction occurs between the instructor and the students using personal computers with Web cameras, microphones, and speakers. There are numerous options available for video conferencing software and

Internet-based tools,[7] such as *Adobe ConnectPro, GoToMeeting,* or *ReadyTalk.* Video conferencing can incorporate the use of white boards that have an interactive space where text, multimedia, Web pages, and applications can be shared between students and faculty.[6] Video conferencing can also be used to conduct virtual office hours where students can make appointments to have private sessions with the course instructor. Video conferencing promotes a sense of connectedness for students, and it can be a mechanism for interaction between students, instructors, and course content.[2] Because video conferencing requires all participants to be online at the same time, it can be challenging to schedule a conference at a time that is convenient for everyone, particularly when course participants live in different time zones or work different shifts.[2]

Chat rooms

Chat rooms with instant messaging are another synchronous method of communication. Conversations are typed in real time, allowing for immediate response and feedback between students and instructors who are online at the same time.

With chat rooms, the ability to participate and contribute to the conversation in a timely fashion can be hampered if a participant is a slow typist. By the time a message is typed and sent, the conversation may well have moved on to another topic.[2]

Asynchronous Courses

Asynchronous courses are also Web based, similar to synchronous courses. However, students' participation occurs at a time and place that is convenient for them and does not require them to be online a specific time or day. The instructor determines the completion deadlines for the graded activities. Communication is time delayed, for example, a required discussion may have a week for the dialogue among students before it is closed. This type of course delivery is well suited to meet the needs of perioperative nurses who are working full time and do not have the time to travel to an onsite course. The often-chaotic schedules in the operating room can make it difficult for perioperative nurses to commit to being present in a virtual classroom at a specific time or on a specific day. Common methods of communication in asynchronous courses are email, electronic bulletin boards and threaded discussion forums, webcasts, and blogs.

E-mail

The use of e-mail can promote a sense of connectedness between students and the instructor.[6] It is a convenient way to communicate when students are accessing email at various times throughout the day and night because of their location or work schedules. In small classes, e-mail communication is easy to monitor. In addition to being used as a means of communication, it can be used to share course documents and other learning resources, such as links to videos and Websites. A disadvantage to using e-mail is that with large classes, it can be time consuming and overwhelming to keep up with reading and responding to large volumes of e-mails. This is especially the case for the instructor. When e-mails are not answered quickly, students can become frustrated and even disengaged, so setting parameters for response time allows both the student and instructor to have a consistent expectation.[2] Another possible disadvantage with e-mail occurs because the intended tone and inflection can be lost in text-only communication, so there are increased opportunities for misunderstanding of meaning.

Discussion Grading Rubric   Name:

Possible %	Discussion Criteria	Satisfactory	Needs Improvement	Poor	Score
30%	Support from Literature	Postings grounded in literature and includes more than two diferent reference citations per discussion board. *(22-30 points)*	Postings grounded in literture and include only 1 reference citation *(17 points)*	No citations *(0 points)*	
30%	Personal & Professional Insights	Contributes unique perspectives or insights gleaned from personal experience or examples from health care field demonstrating applied course knowledge stimulating peer comments. *(26-30 points)*	Demonstrates perspectives but does not or minimum demonstration of applied course knowledge *(23-25 points)*	Post does not reflect personal response or demonstrate applied course knowledge. *(0-22 points)*	
14%	Organization	Presents information in logical, meaningful, and understandable sequence *(13-14 points)*	Required information is present. Information is sometimes unclear and difficult to follow. *(11-12 points)*	Posting is not relevant to discussion questions. Information often is unclear and difficult to follow *(0-10 points)*	
13%	Grammar & Syntax, APA	APA, Grammar, spelling and/or punctuation accurate, or with minimal errors *(12-13 points)*	A few errors in APA, grammar, spelling, and syntax are noted. *(10-11 points)*	APA, Grammar, spelling and/or punctuation contain multiple errors. *(0-9 points)*	
13%	Timeliness & Interactive Dialogue	Provides initial posts early and responds often. Actively stimulates discussion and promotes and enhances peer dialogue with friqent responses to peers. Engages in substantive dialogue in each discussion board. Posts early and often allowing opportunity for peer dialogue. *(12-13 points)*	Provides initial post on time. Meets minimum requirements for substantive responses. *(10-11 points)*	Does not actively engage or respond to peers. Reacts defensively to feedback and/or questions. And/or, posts late or not at all. *(0-9 points)*	
100%				Total Score	0.00

Fig. 1. Threaded discussion example. (*Courtesy of* Dr Joy Don Baker.)

Threaded discussion

Threaded discussion forums are a common means of communication in asynchronous online courses.[6] Typically, the instructor will initiate a discussion forum for the class by posting a topic and criteria intended to guide the student responses. Within the forum, threads, or topics for discussion, can be started either by the instructor or the students who will then post their responses within the appropriate thread. Threads help keep discussions somewhat organized for both the instructor and the students. Discussion forums can promote dialogue among students that might not occur during real-time class discussions. Discussion forums are utilized to engage students in creative and critical thinking and writing about course content and other related topics.[8] They are designed to create a sense of community, connection, and social interaction among students.[6] Students have more time to reflect on the topic, formulate their answers, and edit them before responding because discussion forums are asynchronous (**Fig. 1**).[3] This can be especially beneficial for shy students and for international students who need to first translate the discussion into their own language before posting a response.

For first-time users of discussion forums, it is helpful to know the instructor's expectations or *rules* for posting. Examples of posting rules or guidelines include:

- Minimum/maximum number of required posts per forum or thread
- Deadline for posting first response
- Deadline for posting last response (date forum closes)
- Minimum/maximum words per post
- Requirements for citing references
- Requirements and criteria for replying to other students posts
- Criteria for defining a post as *substantial*
- How the forum will be graded.

A discussion grading rubric is located in **Fig. 2** and addresses how one instructor addresses the guidelines for all graded discussions in her course.

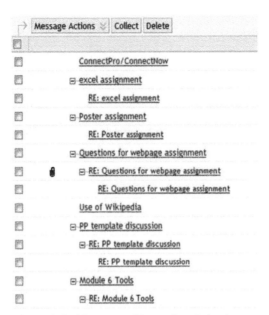

Fig. 2. Discussion grading rubric. (*Courtesy of* Dr Joy Don Baker.)

A disadvantage of discussion forums is that successful dialogue and interaction is dependent on all students' timely participation. If posting parameters are not well established and adhered to, students may wait until the last minute to enter a post, which then makes it difficult for other students to reply. Some students find it inconvenient to have to return to the Website several times throughout the duration of the forum, but it is necessary if responding to other classmates' posts is required.[6]

As a student new to discussion boards, it is helpful to understand the faculty's role in discussion forums. Early on, students may become frustrated that the instructor does not reply to their posts or confirm that their answers are correct. Students may think the instructor is not paying attention or following the conversation when in fact they are delaying their responses to provide more students with the opportunity to post their comments first. To encourage participation, instructors may intentionally ask thought-provoking questions that do not have just one correct answer. Instructors monitor discussions, identify areas of agreement and disagreement, and help students find common ground on divergent issues. They may encourage and recognize a student's contributions to a forum without confirming whether their response is correct.[9] This can be difficult for students who are concrete thinkers and desire affirmation that their answers are right or wrong. It may be helpful for these students to know that the goal of threaded discussion forums is to help students engage in activities that promote critical thinking, collaborative learning, and reflective writing as opposed to simply soliciting correct answers to straightforward questions.[9]

Blogs

Blogs are like discussion forums except access to them expands beyond the environment of a learning management system such as *Blackboard, Angel, or Moodle*. Blogs are Web based and are available for viewing and comment by anyone with access to the blogger's Uniform Resource Locator (URL). In a personal journal–like format, students can post their thoughts, opinions, ideas, and knowledge about a topic of interest, and anyone viewing the blog can post a responding comment. Blogging empowers students to learn by expressing themselves through writing, and because access to the student's blog is available to a broader public forum (not constrained to just their classmates) they may experience global citizenship beyond the classroom.[9]

Wikis

Dawley[6] quotes Wiki founder, Ward Cunningham's definition of wikis as "a collection of Web pages which can be edited by anyone, at any time, from anywhere." One of the more well-known wikis is *Wikipedia*.[10] Another site is the *WikiWikiWeb*[11] that allows wiki participants to engage and add to content about wikis. The key disadvantage to wiki use is that it is constantly changing and is not peer reviewed. However, it can serve as an excellent tool for student group work, and a learning management system such as *Blackboard* offers a wiki course tool that faculty may choose to use within their course.

Webcasts

Webcasts are similar to Webinars, but students are not required to be online at any given time. Webcasts are presentations that are recorded and then made available for students to access at a time that is convenient for them. Webcasts can replace lectures done by course faculty. These may take the format of voiceover *PowerPoint* or capturing videos in software, such as *Captivate* or *Camtasia*.

ENROLLMENT PLANNING

Perioperative nurses who are considering enrolling in an online class for the first time may want to assess their readiness to transition from more traditional face-to-face classroom settings. A student will want to assess whether they possess some of the key characteristics of successful online students[2]: A successful online student will (be):

- A highly motivated, independent, and active learner
- Manage time wisely and be well organized
- Self-motivated and self-disciplined and will take responsibility for their learning
- Willing to adapt to new ways of learning and accept that quality learning can take place outside of the traditional classroom
- Willing to share work, personal experiences, and expertise by working in groups and teams
- Skilled in written communication and be willing to speak up to voice an opinion
- Willing to take constructive criticism from faculty and fellow students
- Willing to participate in activities that promote reflection, critical thinking, and decision making
- Willing to commit 4 to 12 or more hours of study time a week per class.[2]

TECHNOLOGY AND SKILLS

Online classes are technology dependent; therefore, it is critical that students have access to a personal computer with dependable Internet service. Utilizing a work computer may be an option, but for security reasons, many health care institutions limit employees' full access to the Worldwide Web. They may prohibit employees from downloading large files or receiving e-mailed attachments, all of which are necessary in online courses. In addition to having access to computer and to the

Internet, certain technologic skills are required to be successful in an online class.[2] Theses skills include:

- Keyboarding skills
- Basic to intermediate word processing skills (for example Microsoft Word)
- Basic ability to use presentation software (for example Microsoft PowerPoint)
- Ability to send, receive, and manage e-mail
- Ability to attach files to e-mail and open attachments in e-mail
- Basic digital file management skills
- Utilize search engines to find Websites and information on the Worldwide web
- Ability to upload and download files
- Basic use of printer skills.[2]

A perioperative nurse contemplating their readiness to enroll in an online class may also find the Websites listed after the references helpful.

SUMMARY

There is a renewed national focus on advancing the education levels of all nurses. Universities and colleges now offer online nursing courses and degree programs, which makes access to higher levels of education better than ever for perioperative nurses who want to return to school yet continue to work in the operating room. An understanding of the personal characteristics and technologic skills required for successful online learning will guide the decision-making process when considering the different delivery methods of nursing education. In addition to the traditional or face-to-face classroom setting, perioperative nurses have the option to enroll in a hybrid or blended course that may use either or both synchronous and asynchronous content delivery methods within the online course. Knowing the different requirements and characteristics of these delivery methods will assist the perioperative nurse to select the type of course that will best suit their personal lifestyle and learning style and accommodate their professional schedules and meet their educational needs.

REFERENCES

1. Institute of Medicine. Future of Nursing: Leading Change, Advancing Health. 2010. p. 4–15.
2. O'Neil CA, Fisher CA, Newbold SK. Developing online learning environments in nursing education. New York: Springer Publishing Company, LLC; 2009.
3. Johnson AE. A nursing faculty's transition to teaching online. Nursing Education Perspectives 2008;20(1):17–22.
4. Billings DM, Halstead JA. Teaching in nursing: a guide for faculty. 3rd edition. St Louis: Saunders Elsevier; 2009.
5. Schoolcraft V, Novotny J. A nuts-and-bolts approach to teaching nursing. Second ed. Springer Series On The Teaching of Nursing. New York: Springer Publishing Company; 2000.
6. Dawley L. The tools for successful online teaching. Hershey (PA): Information Science Publishing (an imprint of Idea Group inc); 2007. p. 244.
7. Wooley DR. Thinkofit web conferencing review, an independent guide to software for web collaboration, web conferencing, online communities and social media. Available at: http://thinkofit.com/webconf/index.htm#about. Accessed November 12, 2011.
8. Halstead JA, Frank B. Pathways to a nursing education career: Educating the next generation of nurses. New York: Springer Publishing Company; 2011.

9. O'Neil CA, Fisher CA, Newbold SK. Developing an online course: best practices for nurse educators. In: McGivern DO, editor. Springer Series on the Teaching of Nursing. New York: Springer Publishing Company; 2004. p. 69.

10. Wikipedia. Available at: http://www.wikipedia.org/. Accessed September 23, 2011.

11. WikiWikiWeb. Available at: http://www.c2.com/cgi/wiki. Accessed September 16, 2011.

FURTHER READINGS

Penn State University Learning Design Community Hub. Student self-assessment for online learning readiness. Available at: http://ets.tlt.psu.edu/learningdesign/assessment/onlinecontent/online_readiness. Accessed September 19, 2011.

College of DuPage Center for Independent Learning & Instructional Center. Do I have the technical skills? Available at: http://marylandonline.org/assessments/technical-skills. Accessed September 19, 2011.

Roles of the Perioperative Nurse and Informaticist and Implications for Practice, Education, and Administration

Michelle B. Eckhard, RN, MSN[a,b],*, Delores Martin, RN, CNOR, BSN[c]

KEYWORDS

• Informatics • Technology • Perioperative nurse • Practice

KEY POINTS

• Technology within the scope of patient care is advancing.
• Informatics is the specialty of nursing which advances the use of technology within patient care to enhance safety.
• Perioperative nursing informatics is a subspecialty within the nursing informatics role which is experiencing a significant growth.

Technology and innovation are vital partners in the patient safety improvement process. For new innovation and technology to succeed in this process, it must be supported by the nurses who use it, the informaticist who supports it, the educators who ensure it is correctly utilized, the administrators who must budget for it, and the researchers who will demonstrate the value of technological advancements in improving patient safety. Providing training for the use of new equipment and ensuring competency of staff who will use that equipment is one of the roles of the educator, but requiring that training is a role of the administration for the surgical department.

ROLES OF THE PERIOPERATIVE NURSE

Safety is a key concept that is impacted by technology, for both the patient and the staff who use it.[1] Preoperative nurses must utilize the technology provided in the

The authors have nothing to disclose.
[a] Trinity Mother Frances Hospitals and Clinics, 800 East Dawson, Tyler, TX 75701, USA
[b] Graduate Nursing Administration Program, University of Texas at Arlington College of Nursing, Arlington, TX, USA
[c] Surgical Services, Texas Health Presbyterian Hospital, 1105 North Central Expressway Allen, TX 75013, USA
* Corresponding author. Trinity Mother Frances Hospitals and Clinics, 800 East Dawson, Tyler, TX 75701.
E-mail address: EckharM@tmfhs.org

Perioperative Nursing Clinics 7 (2012) 171–175
doi:10.1016/j.cpen.2012.02.003
1556-7931/12/$ – see front matter © 2012 Elsevier Inc. All rights reserved.

manner in which it was designed to ensure their patients' safety and maintain quality patient care. Perioperative nurses use computers for multiple purposes within the operative area, including reviewing the patient electronic medical record. One important area is obtaining laboratory results. Orders placed electronically allow faster turnaround time, allowing laboratory and test results to be viewed by the appropriate perioperative care provider in real time.

Other areas in which technology impacts the perioperative nurse include documentation of care provided, tracking of instruments and staff members, and delivery of medications.[2] Through appropriate use of the many forms of technology available to the perioperative nurse, adverse events, such as administration of the incorrect preoperative antibiotic, can be decreased through the use of bar code medication verification.[2] The practice of the perioperative nurse will continue to grow while incorporating the technology available. The direction that growth will take can be influenced by the willingness of the nurses to get involved, becoming change leaders and activists in the process of enhancing patient safety through planning and utilization of technology. Perioperative nursing documentation is incorporated into the electronic health record (EHR), making that information available in real time to all practitioners who have been granted access to the record. One practitioner who would use this information is the pathologist who examines specimens removed during the surgery. The nurses involved in the use of the equipment are key to ensuring that other perioperative professionals receive proper training on equipment.

A new specialty within the nursing informaticist role is developing, which focuses on the perioperative nurse's use of technology. As new technology is created, software vendors combine perioperative nurses' experience with science to develop products with practical application to the role of the perioperative nurse.[2]

Another developing role is the Master's Prepared Perioperative Advance Practice Nurse (APN) degree. A nurse with this degree provides care for surgical patients and their families throughout the perioperative process. This practitioner prevents delays in surgery cases by assessing patients and reviewing their histories and providing information to the surgeon and anesthesia provider through documentation into the EHR, which may influence a positive outcome for the patient. Through reviewing information within the EHR, this perioperative APN can identify any preoperative tests or procedures that were not completed that could have caused a delay in the case. After evaluating the information, this APN can inform the surgical team of anything that may influence how the surgical care is provided for that patient, especially if research is necessary to clarify unusual diseases processes.[2] This APN can also identify educational and emotional needs the patient may have related to the surgery.

ROLE OF THE INFORMATICIST

Nursing has embraced technology to improve patient care for decades.[3] The field of nursing is evolving from low to high technology. The role of nursing informatics has developed to serve as a bridge between nursing and technology. The Nurse Informaticist utilizes nursing knowledge to ensure that appropriate software, hardware, and equipment choices are made. They assist with implementation of new technology and provide ongoing support of software and equipment. Their technology background allows them to identify optimization opportunities related to the technology used by the perioperative clinical staff. Additionally, informaticists utilize their clinical background to identify the need for appropriate technology and equipment to meet the requirements of the jobs, such as selection of electronic tablets to document with the EHR rather than a large desktop computer within the operating room to allow the nurse to have her documentation readily available, regardless of where she is in the perioperative suite. This enhances the practice of nursing through the use of informatics. Nurse informatics specialists must embrace innovation and use technology that advances nursing care and enriches the profession.[3]

One role of the informaticist is to provide tools that allow perioperative staff to identify improvements in patient care through analysis of data related to patient outcomes.[4] Analysis of that data helps drive care decisions based on the evidence derived and builds the bank of evidence-based practice models. Mobile applications have been developed to track process workflow within the perioperative arena to investigate how different types of care provided affects patient flow through the operating room (OR).[5] Analysis of these data by the informatics nurse can provide benchmarking and simulations. This can be used to determine a flow map to identify causes of delays while increasing the efficiency of staffing within the OR. The role of the perioperative informatics nurse specialist has evolved as technology within the perioperative area has grown.[2] These specialists become certified as system administrators for the systems used within the OR. Other specialties for informatics nurses within the perioperative area are nurse educators, robotics specialists, and research consultants. Nurses can also work for companies that provide the technology, helping companies choose the appropriate equipment and technology because of a shared knowledge of the perioperative workflow.[2]

IMPLICATIONS FOR PRACTICE

Technology has increased the proficiency of the nursing profession. Charting is now completed on the computer.[6] Physicians enter orders into the computer system, resulting in a decrease in medication errors due to poor penmanship.[1] Medication orders are available to the pharmacy for verification as soon as the physician enters the orders in the computer. All care providers are able to view the laboratory results more quickly because of the advancement in technology implemented with the EHR.

Changes to surgery techniques within the last few decades meant changes for the circulating nurse. Computer charting is more prevalent in the OR. The circulating nurse can place orders in the computer for laboratory results on specimens, which decreases the time needed to obtain results. Currently, surgery involving robotics includes laparoscopic gallbladder surgery and appendectomy and arthroscopic procedures such as partial and total joint replacement. Circulating nurses need to be proficient and knowledgeable in the use of equipment for these types of surgery to ensure equipment is correctly set up and operating for the procedure.[2] As the technology within the operating room increases, so does the need for advanced training among the circulating nurses. Additional roles of nursing informatics within the operating room arena are being developed, which include perioperative robotics nurse specialists, supply company representatives, research consultants to track best outcomes, and evidence-based practices. Patients are benefiting from this type of procedure because of smaller incisions, shorter hospitalizations, and faster healing with fewer complications.

IMPLICATIONS FOR EDUCATION

Nurses currently in practice bring a wide range of technological savvy to the workplace.[7] Depending on their previous experience and education, veteran nurses may have limited computer technology literacy. Equipment within health care settings varies from one facility to another. This creates a challenge for academic educators who must provide current, relevant content to students to ensure they have adequate skills to utilize equipment they will find within the workplace. Eley and colleagues[7] report that of the 10,000 nurses surveyed about the information technology and training they had received, 83% report they use computers as part of their workflow. Half of these nurses reported that the training they had received as part of their employment was insufficient to meet the computer and technology aspect of their jobs. These nurses also reported a feeling that their career development was hampered by their lack of technology skills.

This gap in skill is amplified when a nurse returns to the perioperative setting after an extended time away. The challenge for educators is to assess the competency level of each nurse and develop a training plan to ensure correct use of technology. Orientation for new perioperative nurses must focus on the specific equipment each staff member will be working with and can be extended to ensure competency.[2] With the advancement of operative technology, perioperative nurses may specialize in specific types of surgeries, such as orthopedic or robotic. As technology continues to advance the practice of nursing, educators must incorporate this into the nursing curricula to ensure new nurses have updated information and skills to utilize the new technology. Perioperative nurse educators within hospital settings must also develop methods of maintaining competency standards and evaluations for staff nurses. Mock ORs are being used as one method of training and testing nurses' competencies, focusing on equipment and instruments that will be utilized within the OR.[2]

As the technology within the OR advances, the need for continuous training of the staff increases.[2] Basic nursing knowledge is not sufficient for a perioperative nurse to function within today's OR, and nursing education programs struggle to keep up with technology new nurses will face on the job. Training within the OR for new equipment may be conducted by the sale representatives, which may require hands-on training and time commitment away from the unit. Orientation of new nurses may take up to 9 months to ensure they are competent with equipment such as laparoscopic towers, robots, and the EHR, technology that they must work with on a daily basis.

IMPLICATIONS FOR ADMINISTRATION

Implementing technology by replicating paper processes to an electronic format does not ensure successful or appropriate utilization of technology.[1] Inappropriate or incorrect utilization of technology can actually hamper patient safety rather than enhance it. Any introduction of technology creates change within a culture and must be supported by the administration. Strategic planning that defines the need for change, scope, and recognition of the impact of that change is necessary to ensure success for technology projects. Costs that must be calculated into the budget include not only the cost of the equipment but also the training to ensure safe operation by the staff within the operating room.

Administrators must ensure that key people who make decisions related to technology as well as nursing informaticists are employed for this purpose. Ensuring that informaticians are utilized to the benefit of both the practitioner and the hospital is one of the roles administrators play.[8] Informaticians must be allowed to use their knowledge of the art and science of nursing to ensure proper equipment, software, and hardware purchase choices are made. Costs of technology increase with each version of software, and hardware is quickly outdated. Introduction of technology creates change in processes and sometimes the culture of an organization and often makes things seem worse before they become better.[1] A well-defined strategy and recognition of the impact of the change on the people involved are necessary for a successful technology initiative. Administrators must ensure that budgeting for technology must include sufficient funding for training with each implementation to ensure staff competence. Staff that is well trained to use the new technology is essential for the success of the new technology.

SUMMARY

Technological advances continue to present options to enhance patient safety. One small piece of technology, the EHR, alerts the perioperative nurse and physicians to potential problems that could occur with medications or with the patient's care. The challenge for health care providers is to maintain a balance, ensuring staff can depend on the equipment provided without forfeiting the utilization of critical thinking skills. Administrators play a key role in ensuring the right people are in place to choose the appropriate software, hardware, and technology equipment to ensure decisions are made wisely, keeping in mind safety, cost, and efficiency. Technology within all fields of nursing is advancing at a rapid rate. Perioperative nurses, as well as all nurses, must be involved in that evolution, doing their part to advance the practice of nursing through the proper use of technology.

REFERENCES

1. Simpson RL. Patient and nurse safety: how information technology makes a difference. Nurs Adm Q 2005;29(1):97–101.
2. Sweeney P. The effects of information technology on perioperative nursing. AORN J 2010; 92(5):528–40.
3. Parker PJ. One nurse informatics specialist views the future: technology in the crystal ball. Nurs Adm Q 2005;29(2):123–4.
4. Carters K. Nursing informatics, outcomes and quality improvement. AACN Clinical Issues 2003;14(3):283–94.
5. Hynh N, Taafee K, Fredendall L, et al. The use of a mobile application to track process workflow in perioperative services. Comput Inform Nurs 2011;29(6):368–74.
6. Struk C, Moss J. Focus on technology: what can you do to move the vision forward? Comput Inform Nurs 2009;29(5):192–6.
7. Eley R, Fallon T, Soar J, et al. The status of training and education in information and computer technology of Australian nurses: a national survey. J Clin Nurs 2008;17: 2758–67.
8. McLane S, Turley J. Informaticians: how they may benefit your healthcare organization. J Nurs Adm 2011;41(1):29–35.

Cyber Diving:
Information Searching

Helen Hough, MLS, BS, BA

KEYWORDS

- Web pages • Information resource evaluation • Information management • Internet
- Decision making

KEY POINTS

- Formal analysis of a research problem can help structure a literature search.
- Different Internet search engines have many useful features for focusing the search.
- Understanding the provenance of documents also focuses the search.
- Search engines and literature databases use special commands called Boolean operators to combine search terms.
- Using these techniques when searching in Internet search engines, Google Scholar, and specialized databases including PubMed, CINAHL, and PsycInfo yields excellent results.
- In addition to immediate full-text or purchase there are several other options that perioperative nurses can use to obtain discovered resources.

As health care providers, we want to be able to provide the best care to our patients. Occasionally we observe that some caring process may not be the most effective it could or should be. Some of these processes are direct patient interactions, disease prevention, and intervention, but the idea of best care can be related to the timeliness and cost of that care. Best care is based on evidence indicating that the care provided is the best that can be done and that it is done at the most appropriate level. This evidence is derived through research and expert consensus efforts. The evidence is then documented and published so it can be disseminated to the health care providers who need it. Continuing education is one way of renewing our knowledge and discovering some of the most common methods of providing quality care. When questions arise related to a specific local provision of care, a person may need to create the time to investigate these perceived problems. Sharing the solutions through inservice, teaching, and writing for publication can also benefit others outside of an immediate practice and thereby improve care for all.

The author has nothing to disclose.
Science and Engineering Library, University of Texas at Arlington, PO Box 19497, B03 Nedderman Hall, 416 Yeats Street, Arlington, TX 76019, USA
E-mail address: hough@uta.edu

Perioperative Nursing Clinics 7 (2012) 177–188
doi:10.1016/j.cpen.2012.02.009
1556-7931/12/$ – see front matter © 2012 Elsevier Inc. All rights reserved.

A literature search is done when information is needed to properly address a perceived problem. The literature search may be easy because something needs to be confirmed, for example, looking up a laboratory value to confirm that the patient's test result is too high or too low. Sometimes the problem is more complex and finding the answer is not as easy as using a standard reference tool. A simple literature search can occasionally easily find a resource because a more complex problem has already been addressed by the work done by others and has been made freely available. Sometimes a fee is required to access a discovered resource.

Sometimes the information found was developed long enough ago that additional information has rendered the previous response inappropriate. Even if the information is timely something about the study setting or patient group may not be relevant to the current situation. In these cases, we discover that we may have a new or specific question that still needs to be investigated. The literature review can then provide guidance related to the level of knowledge deficit and the amount of new information to be developed. That said, many people find that the discovery process will take much longer than expected. As an example, how long does it really take to confirm the outside levels of a lab value? Whereas it may take a second or two to actually find the value, the real time spent should include the time spent finding the right phone number of the person who might have the data or locating the document or program containing the data. Even the time to walk to where the resource should be considered. Fortunately, time locating the resource may be reduced by asking a colleague who might know the location of the document. For a more complex problem requiring a complex literature review, guess an amount of time you are willing to spend, then assume it will take four times longer. Often how the problem is framed may cause delays, or other issues may arise in the search process. Discuss the problem with a couple of colleagues for ideas on how to frame the question, set up the literature research protocol, and then start searching. If the total search takes less than the projected extended period, feel free to be proud of the skills you exhibited.

A good literature review can be started without considering costs associated with access to the discovered materials. The search process itself is also independent of a detailed analysis of the resources located. Once appropriate and sufficient material is identified, then issues related to obtaining the best subset of these resources can be considered.

HOW TO SEARCH

A high quality literature search requires several kinds of problem-solving behaviors to successfully identify, locate, and use the materials. Searching is a fairly linear sequence of problem solving because the literature is heavily computerized. Computer programs can only retrieve what is related to what is entered; these programs do not guess what the user wants or means. The process begins with the analysis of the problem and developing query terminology that will be understandable to the relevant computer systems. Taking the time at the very beginning to set up the question for the computer will speed the search process. During the search, the search strategy may need to be adjusted based on information discovered during the earlier part of the search. Documenting the search strategy and steps is critical because search reiteration with new or alternate terms is reasonable and should be expected. Documentation of efforts already completed reduces unnecessary duplication.

Initially gather more information than absolutely necessary. After the search is mostly completed, analyze the gathered materials to select the most appropriate. The mechanical process of obtaining the documents can be done partly during the search process and partly after the search is completed. The final, and most fulfilling, part of the literature review should be the how the materials are used.

FRAME THE QUESTION

Most health care problems can be translated into a clinical question and then a research question. I often explain that the research question is similar to a diagnostic investigation. The diagnostician takes a history, which leads to a guess at the reasons for the problem and then proceeds to determine if this guess is correct. The evidence provided by laboratory tests will determine the correct diagnosis. The diagnosis then informs the clinician of appropriate treatments for the problem. The question format allows us to better break the issue into the components needed to be investigated. The patient's health care problem of a fever turns into the common clinical question of, "Why does the patient have this fever," and the associated diagnostic (research) question might be, "Does this patient have the flu." The subsequent tests are a linear process of discovering if there are indications of a viral infection. Some tests may even be done in order to eliminate a bacterial infection. A literature review is similar; there is a clinical question, there is a research question, and there are various investigative tools in order to develop a diagnosis and eventually the correct treatment.

The example used throughout this discussion begins with the problem of the cost of cleaning scrubs. Of course, a quick response could be to simply change the process from having the hospital send the scrubs out to be cleaned to requiring all personnel to provide their own scrubs. As tempting as this thought may be, there may be a clinical problem of infection control. The clinical problem could be, "Is there a difference in cost and efficacy when the scrubs are cleaned at home as opposed to when the scrubs are cleaned by hospital vendors." Breaking this clinical question into its conceptual components is the next step in the analysis of the question.

DIVIDE THE QUESTION

Divide the question into conceptual units. Think about the concepts within the question. The computer systems we use do not understand the meaning of a full sentence; the programs are responding to the sequence of words. Most computer systems will attempt to identify materials that match all of the words used in a query. If too many words or terms are used, the computer system will have difficulty in locating materials. Computer systems do not usually understand prepositions; they only match letters and do not understand the idea of terms like *before*, *under*, and *for*. They often also have difficulty responding to verbs. The most effective response from a query is achieved by forming the query into enough words that correspond to the question but no more. Effective search phrases are not in sentence form but are rather in phrases that describe the concepts within the question. Based on the author's experience, most research questions are composed of at least three concepts. Often these concepts can be in the form of nouns. There are several concepts within the question of cost and efficacy of scrub cleaning methods. The focus of the question is specifically the hospital clothing, the *scrubs*. Another concept is *cleaning,* which can be set as the noun, *clean*. Setting aside the cost of cleaning, perhaps a more important concept within this question is the idea of *efficacy,* or *effective*. Additional concepts are *home* and *vendors,* although if we think about it, who else would be cleaning scrubs? If there are only two alternatives, perhaps it is not necessary to include these concepts in the first round of the search. On initial analysis there are three major concepts: (a) scrubs, (b) clean, and (c) efficacy.

This technique is similar to PICO, a framework in evidence-based health care and used by health care researchers and practitioners.[1] PICO was developed as a method to analyze clinical questions for effective, efficient literature retrieval. PICO emphases

Table 1 PICO documentation			
Clinical Problem: Cost of cleaning scrubs			
Research Question: Is there a difference in cost and efficacy when the scrubs are cleaned at home as opposed to when the scrubs are cleaned by hospital vendors			
	Population	Intervention	Outcome
	Scrubs	*Cleaning*	*Efficacy*
Alternative Terms/Synonyms	Clothing Uniforms	Laundering/laundered Washing	Contamination Microorganisms Infectioncontrol

Abbreviation: PICO, population, intervention, comparison, outcome.

patient problem or population (P), intervention (I), comparison (C), and outcome(s) (O) as conceptual units. PICO and PIO (patient, intervention and outcome) have been standards for structuring inquiries for evidence-based practice since the early 1990s. These methods became standards because they work well. Effective, experienced literature searchers tend to incorporate the PICO structure without conscious effort. Additional insights about the PICO method can be found in current books about evidence-based medicine and online from medical libraries.

SYNONYMS WITHIN THE CONCEPTS

Our question does not have a specific patient group but does have a *population*, scrubs, to which an *intervention*, cleaning, will be applied. The question is also examining the *outcome* of efficacy, so PICO/PIO is a reasonable framework (**Table 1**). We can use these three words in an Internet search and there will be Web pages that display. A simple search of "efficacy clean scrubs" in *Google* yields over 500,000 records; *Yahoo*, over 130,000; and *Bing*, over 125,000 records. Many of those Web pages will be about vendors who want the hospital cleaning business. Others are about surgical cleaning methods. Reviewing and discarding all the irrelevant materials is not an effective use of time. In addition, there may be alternative terms that are used by the authors of the preferred type of literature not yet discovered. A little rumination may also lead to the conclusion that scrubs are in the class of clothing. A brief examination of chanced-upon relevant news sources will yield useful synonyms.[2]

Using an Internet search engine is a fine way to start and may or may not be the best way to end. Testing the discovered synonyms in a preferred search engine will help in determining when to stop. "Clothing laundered contamination" as an alternate search phrase yields interesting results (**Table 2**), and the suggestion of adding a modifier, hospital, is appropriate.

HOW INTERNET SEARCH ENGINES IDENTIFY RESOURCES

When the modifier is added to an Internet search query, the number of search results increases relative to the unmodified search. This is because most Internet search engines first retrieve results that have all the terms most often, then the documents that have the terms near each other, followed by documents that have some of the terms but not all. Consequently, the more words one uses with an Internet search engine, the larger and less focused the retrieval becomes. Examining the search engine's help pages will provide information about the

Table 2
Internet search results

Exact Strategy	Internet Search Engine	Approximate Records	Observations
Is there a difference in cost and efficacy when the scrubs are cleaned at home as opposed to when the scrubs are cleaned by hospital vendors?	Google	1,000,000	Imprecise: hand scrubs, vacuum cleaners, etc
	Yahoo	190,000	Imprecise: hospital-focused but still imprecise (VBACs, cochlear implants, blogs)
	Bing	171,000	Similar to Yahoo results
Clothing Laundered Contamination	Google	1,500,000	Includes pesticide or asbestos contamination
	Yahoo	103,000	Includes pesticide contamination
	Bing	68,000	Hospital-focused results, many commercial sites
Hospital Clothing Laundered Contamination	Google	2,700,000	Hospital-focused results, many educational and commercial sites
	Yahoo	73,000	Hospital-focused results, many commercial sites
	Bing	70,000	Hospital-focused results, many commercial sites
+Hospital +Clothing +Laundered +Contamination[a]	Google (+)	145,000	Hospital-focused results, many educational and commercial sites
	Yahoo (+)	23,000	Hospital-focused results, many commercial sites
	Bing	22,400	Hospital-focused results, many commercial sites

[a] The + immediately before a search term indicates the term MUST be included in each of the retrieved items.

techniques that can be used in that engine to ensure all terms are included and thus focus the results.

ADVANCED SEARCH FEATURES

Using the advanced features of the search engine can help to organize the search so the synonyms are used effectively. The three concepts now have three or four synonyms each and possible setting modifiers of hospital *OR* clinical (**Table 3**).

Table 3 PIO results		
Population	**Intervention**	**Outcome**
(a) Hospital *OR* Clinical	Cleaning *OR* Laundering	Efficacy *OR* Contamination
(b) Scrubs *OR* Clothing *OR* Uniforms	*OR* Washing	*OR* Microorganisms *OR* Infection control

Abbreviation: PIO, patient, intervention, outcome.

ORGANIZATIONS DISSEMINATING INFORMATION

Consider the kinds of organizations or agencies that might be addressing parts of the question. If raw data are needed, what agency collects these data, or would the data be likely from a research study? If the question has been studied, then would the results be published in journal literature? It the question is related to a standardized protocol or guideline, which organization or association would be interested in this kind of process? Using search engines' advanced search features to limit to organization or government Web sites is a simple matter of realizing and using the Domain Name System (DNS) conventions. Web addresses are composed of distinct parts and often look something like http://xxx.yyyyyyy.zzz. The third section after the two slashes can be used to identify the type of organization with that Web address.[3] When the organization is an U.S. government agency, this ending can be .gov. If the Web site is part of a more general organization or association, the last component may be .org. US postsecondary educational institutions may use the ending .edu. Countries other than the United States will have an additional section identifying the country of origin. Use the search engine's advanced search features to search within a site or domain with an appropriate domain name ending, for example, a search in *Google* structured as *cleaning hospital clothing site:.gov* will locate material on US government Web sites that have the three words *cleaning*, *hospital*, and *clothing*.

LOCATING TYPES OF MATERIAL

With the number of Internet retrievals that can occur, also consider the kind of materials needed. Types of literature can include journal articles, reviews, systematic reviews, protocols, guidelines, standards, and many others. Professional associations and government agencies may produce useful reports. Many researchers are affiliated with colleges and universities. If data are needed, consider who collects these data. Some data are collected by government agencies including census, population health, and some health care coverage data. Other data are collected by associations, for example US hospital information may be collected by the American Hospital Association, and the American Nurses Association may aggregate data about nurses. Internet search engines have the ability to limit to government, organization, and educational sites if these sites have the Internet addresses that indicate the type of structure.

QUALITY OF INFORMATION

Another consideration is the quality of information needed. High quality information should to be used in developing a resolution to a high-impact problem. Evaluate online resources in a manner similar to evaluating any other kind of resource. First, determine who wrote it or what agency sponsored it. Reliability of the information provider is key. Many businesses will include, as part of their marketing, newsletters and information brochures. These newsletters and brochures can be helpful when the information does not need to be well-documented or is used to provide leads to discovering more about how to find what is needed. Depending on the quality of the writing, these types of resources can also provide overviews of the problem under consideration, terminology used when discussing the issues, and names of people and organizations that investigate aspects of the problem.

Infection control is probably foremost when considering our question of the efficacy of different methods of cleaning hospital uniforms. Thinking broadly, various government agencies and associations are associated with quality information, such as The US Center for Medicaid and Medicare, the US Centers for Disease Control and Prevention, European Centre for Disease Prevention and Control, the Association for Professionals in Infection Control and Epidemiology, the UK National Institute for Health and Clinical Excellence, and so forth. Research grants from these organizations also fund studies that are published in reputable journals.

Thinking broadly about where the needed information may be located allows quick review of sources that may not have the precise focus desired but may provide hints on how to proceed. Colleagues may know of approachable experts who are studying a similar issue. Just as colleagues can be consulted, the references used in a highly related work can also be traced. Protocols found via the US National Guideline Clearinghouse[4] can be used as leads to more focused literature. Systematic reviews from the journal literature, the Cochrane Library, and the Joanna Briggs Institute can be useful for discovering who is publishing within the same topic area.

TOOLS

The Internet can be searched broadly by using one of a variety of freely available search engines. These include *Google*,[5] *Yahoo*,[6] and *Bing*,[7] as well as others. A quick decision on the best search engine to use can be made by repeating the same simple query with a couple of these different Internet search engines and spending a few minutes quickly examining the quantity and quality of the results. Once this decision is made, a quick investigation of the chosen engine's advanced search features will help formulate a precision search. A brief example of how to use a concept's synonyms has already been provided. The search operator **AND** links concepts, and the operator **OR** selects among synonyms. A visual representation of the idea of **AND** and **OR** is shown in **Fig. 1** with the use of Venn diagrams. Most Internet search engines assume an **AND** between any two words unless some other operator is provided.

Using a general search engine may not be efficient if a scholarly review of the literature is needed. If particular types of resources are needed, go immediately to a database that collects information about that kind of resource (books or journal articles). The goal at this point is to discover if an appropriate resource exists. It does not matter if a search engine can provide full text with a click or the database has the resource immediately available. A resource can be obtained if it is known to exist.

Good Web sites for locating books include *Google Books*,[8] *Amazon*,[9] the library book locator *WorldCat*,[10] and bookseller sites. *Google Books* and *Amazon* frequently have book chapters or parts of chapters free for viewing on the Internet. Sometimes these chapters provide excellent leads to researchers and research trends. *WorldCat* is particularly useful for people who have access to a variety of libraries and are not willing to purchase the identified materials. Once a resource is identified within *WorldCat*, a list of libraries by distance from a specific zip code can be displayed. Many libraries including public libraries have a service called interlibrary loan, where

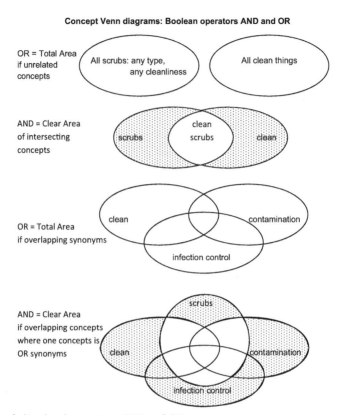

Fig. 1. Search (Boolean) operators *AND* and *OR*.

one library borrows a book from another library for the benefit of a client. Often this service has a minimal cost or is free. Each library system can provide details about an available interlibrary loan service at a library and who may use it.

Journal literature and other research resources can be located by using databases, which aggregate information about these kinds of resources. A commonly known one is produced and distributed by the US National Library of Medicine, *PubMed*.[11] It is one of the most scholarly medical databases, covers all fields of medicine from AIDS to zoology, and includes information about biomedicine, clinical care, research, and health care administration literature. *PubMed* can be easily searched using general keywords, but it also has a standardized vocabulary, which is used to describe its materials. Although not full-text itself, it can provide links to where the full text can be obtained, usually the publisher's site. People associated with many libraries and research institutions have access to additional subscription databases including *CINAHL, PsycINFO, Biological Abstracts*, and the systematic review databases, among others. *CINAHL,* an abbreviation for what used to be the Cumulative Index to Nursing and Allied Health Literature, is designed for nurses and people in related fields and describes nursing and related literature. *PsycINFO* is a database designed for scholars interested in psychology and psychiatry literature. *Biological Abstracts* covers materials focused on biology, zoology, genetics, and so on. All of these databases describe both unique materials as well as those that may be included in other databases. The question devised by the searcher dictates which database should be used first. If the question is generally medical, *PubMed* is an excellent first resource. If the question is nursing-focused, *CINAHL* may be a better first choice. Consult the librarian at a specific institution for a selection of appropriate databases available at that institution. If the searcher selects a particular database or search engine simply based on familiarity, it may not be the best tool to use.

These subscription databases often focus on materials related to specific disciplines of study. These specialized databases may include standardized vocabulary useful to people in these disciplines. Searches within databases like *PubMed* and the subscription databases are examining the description of the materials and not the full text of materials, even though the database may include full text or links to the full text. Sometimes searcher-generated keywords are excellent choices to use as search terms. Sometimes these keywords need to be supplemented with the database-specific standardized search terms. Good literature databases will have well-structured thesauri, and terms will have been assigned to specific articles by skilled people, called indexers, who have read the articles. These terms may be common across databases or limited to specific databases; in either case, observing, using, and recording these terms can add precision to any given search.

Unlike general Internet search engines, subscription databases usually only identify materials that include all search terms used and only when the search phrase exactly matches those in the database. If a searcher enters a search phrase that includes a term not used within a database, nothing is retrieved. Using an uncommon or nonstandard term or an abbreviation will also reduce the quality of the results. Many people attempt to adjust these poor results by adding an additional term, but even less will then be retrieved because all elements of the search are still unfulfillable. Using operators like **AND** and **OR** and combining searcher keywords with the standardized vocabulary usually yields the most robust results. Planning a search strategy and reading some of the help pages can save time in the long run. Being willing to quickly modify a strategy with terminology, specifically standardized vocabulary, is an effective method of obtaining the best results.

Google Scholar[12] is an excellent resource to identify journal articles, books, research reports, and other academic or research-related materials. Its basic search is similar to a general Internet search engine, but the results are limited to relatively scholarly materials. People who are searching *Google Scholar* can also use its advanced search features to limit to specific authors, dates, and broad subject categories, even within specific journals. Its Preferences options include the ability for the searcher to limit to specific languages, limit to types of materials, permit downloading to appropriate bibliographic management software, and identify specific libraries that may have the identified materials. The advantage of *Google Scholar* is that the entire full text can be searched for specific keywords. Its disadvantage is that the keywords may identify material of little relevancy.

As any good searcher knows, checking the references in the back of a resource can lead to additional useful resources. Of course, these resources are older than the item in hand because that author had to read these older works in order to write the article or book. There are tools that can identify resources that have cited a specific document, thereby coming forward in time from the known item. These cited reference searches, based on high quality known works, are much like consulting experts in the field and discovering who else is interested in the same areas and what has been written about them. Most authors of related studies will refer back to a small set of similar or seminal studies, and these studies are commonly cited across the related studies.

Early cited reference searching was done by using the print *Science Citation Index* (SCI) and its related indices.[13] This set of related citation-focused indexes is now distributed electronically as the subscription database, *ISI Web of Knowledge* (WOK). Many academic libraries have access to some or all the covered years. Among other things, WOK analyzes and identifies the relationship between studies based on the common citations between them. It includes the citation information from articles within a relatively small set of high quality journals.

Many other subscription databases, including *CINAHL* and *PsycINFO*, have a cited reference feature. This feature within each of the databases is limited to the references used in articles also within the database. This limitation can be very good because it results in identifying resources of interest to the database developer's targeted audience. The disadvantage is that only the materials selected by the database developer are identified. If the full text can be searched, reference searching can also be done by key phrase searching. Care has to be taken because there are several different citation styles, and searching for an author's full first name may not yield those items where the author's initials have been used as part of a citation.

Because full text should include the references within the text, cited reference searching is relatively easy to do in the broader digital environment with the aforementioned care. However, *Google Scholar* also has a *Cited By* search feature that allows the searcher more leeway. After a search is completed, below each relevant record is a *Cited By* link. Clicking this link will display those items that include the initial item as a cited reference. Precision can be increased by searching for specific keywords within this list by using the check box labeled "Search within articles citing . . . ."

OBTAINING NEEDED DOCUMENTS

The ease of Internet searching when a document displays with a click of a link is wonderful. Care must be taken when looking at these documents. Some free documents do not contain reliable information. The time and effort of developing reliable resources is expensive. Organizations also incur continuing costs when maintaining access to these resources. As a result of these costs, many of the reliable resources will require a purchase fee. Fortunately, many authors and organizations, because of their concern for scholarship and the transmission of knowledge, have adopted the Open Access philosophy and have work posted in their institutional repositories. These repositories are usually associated with educational or government institutions and are Internet-accessible. In an Internet search, checking alternate listings for the same document may be worthwhile. The official form of a published article, together with any online enhancements, may still be the publisher's Web site, but some pre- or postreview manuscripts may be available on other sites. The contract between the author and the publisher determines if an author can post a copy and, when possible, which version.

OPTIONS BESIDES PAYING ONLINE

There are additional options if instant access is not required. Many people are unaware of the various services that exist to support evidence-based health care. Some of these opportunities and services are available through colleagues, professional organizations, and libraries. Research services may include access to collections that already contain needed documents, access to subscription services with full-text resources, or ability to order materials at a lower cost than independent online purchases.

Networking with colleagues is important. The support from peers, from working through ideas to finding materials, is valuable. Professional nurses and scholars will subscribe to professional journals and other services. A hospital nurse can ask colleagues interested the field of study if they have a specific document. Beyond the hospital, nurses may find useful information from their professional organizations. Many organizations also have libraries and other support services for their members. An examination of these organizations' Web sites or a phone call may lead to many valuable resources.

Just as health care is provided in more places than only hospitals, not all hospitals provide the same services, and more than just nurses and doctors work in hospitals, so also information is available through more than just the Internet. Many hospital networks also have good libraries and library services. These institutional libraries exist to support the efforts of the people who work for the institution. The librarians and other library staff members can provide valuable assistance in the research processes. Many resources may already be available to the perioperative nurse who calls or visits the library. If the hospital is affiliated with a college, university, or other educational institution, the staff and services of the institutional library can be supportive of the nurse. Local public libraries are also very useful. Public libraries exist to support the needs of the members of the community. The members of the community include residents and businesses. Services in these different kinds of libraries can include assistance in the question development and search strategy phases. Different databases and support in using these resources may be available. Collections of useful resources and methods of obtaining additional resources are among the many services libraries provide.

The US National Library of Medicine (NLM) is the largest medical library in the world. The mission of this library is to enable biomedical research, support health care and public health, and promote healthy behavior.[14] Among many other things, the NLM is the creator of *PubMed*, the medical database available worldwide. American health care providers, through the National Network of Libraries of Medicine, have access to NLM resources and more (http://nnlm.gov/). Many other countries have similar national medical libraries and library systems that assist their health care providers and support the health of their citizens.

SUMMARY

The Internet provides easy access to a lot of information. Although access is easy, finding the most appropriate information in a timely fashion can be difficult. Analyzing the research question is the first step in finding information effectively and efficiently. The search process is a discovery process, and one of the last steps may be actually retrieving identified resources. The identified resources may be available online or through a variety of library and other information services.

A complex literature search may require several different combinations of thinking styles and search iterations to retrieve substantive materials. There are many ways to discover appropriate information, from using keywords and standardized terminology to using the references within the documents as part of the discovery process. Understanding the differences between various Internet search engines and being aware of their advanced search features is useful. Specialized techniques can be used to create precise search queries. Search precision can also be increased by using subject-focused databases, some of which are available over the Internet and others through library support services.

As with any skill, practice and familiarity will improve search efficacy. When stumbling through a literature search, it may be comforting to remember that no one will die from these stumbles, nor will the Internet accidentally break. When asked, colleagues and librarians can help both novice and expert searchers at any point of the literature search processes. This literature provides the opportunities for evidence-based practice. Perioperative registered nurses who engage in evidence-based practice improve the health care provided to many people. Nurses who share their knowledge of searching and locating this evidence empower other providers to improve health care even more.

REFERENCES

1. Richardson WS, Wilson MC, Nishikawa J, et al. The well-built clinical question: a key to evidence-based decisions. ACP J Club 1995;123:A12–13.
2. Hospital scrubs are a dangerous fashion statement. Infection Control Today 2008, December 3. Available at: http://www.infectioncontroltoday.com/news/2008/12/hospital-scrubs-are-a-dangerous-fashion-statement.aspx. Accessed February 19, 2012.
3. Internet Corporation for Assigned Names and Numbers. Root Zone Database. Available at: http://www.iana.org/domains/root/db/. Accessed February 19, 2012.
4. Agency for Healthcare Research and Quality. National Guideline Clearinghouse. Available at: http://www.guideline.gov/. Accessed February 19, 2012.
5. Google [search engine]. Available at: http://www.google.com. Accessed February 19, 2012.
6. Yahoo [search engine]. Available at: http://www.yahoo.com. Accessed February 19, 2012.
7. Bing [search engine]. Available at: http://www.bing.com. Accessed February 19, 2012.
8. Google. Google Books [search engine books; includes many excerpts and full text]. Available at: http://www.google.com/books. Accessed February 19, 2012.
9. Amazon [merchandize distributor]. Available at: http://amazon.com. Accessed February 19, 2012.
10. OCLC Online Computer Library Center, Inc. WorldCat [aggregated library catalogs]. Available at: http://www.worldcat.org. Accessed February 19, 2012.
11. US National Library of Medicine. PubMed [biomedical literature database]. Available at: http://www.pubmed.gov. Accessed February 19, 2012.
12. Google. Google Scholar [search engine for scholarly literature; focuses on articles and patents but may identify research reports, books, and more]. Available at: http://www.google.com/books. Accessed February 19, 2012.
13. Thomson Reuters. History of citation indexing. Available at: http://thomsonreuters.com/products_services/science/free/essays/history_of_citation_indexing/. Accessed February 19, 2012.
14. US National Library of Medicine. The National Library of Medicine (Fact Sheet). Available at: http://www.nlm.nih.gov/pubs/factsheets/nlm.html. Accessed February 19, 2012.

Evaluating Website Resources

Helen Hough, MLS, BS, BA

KEYWORDS

- Webpages • Information resource evaluation • Information management • Internet
- Decision making

KEY POINTS

- The evaluation of websites can be made easier by using relevancy and reliability criteria.
- The contents of webpages are relevant when they meet the needs of the viewers in terms of content purpose, coverage, language, and timeliness.
- Reliability can be assessed when there is information about the author and hosting site along with contact data, good spelling and grammar, and the date of creation.
- Most importantly, viewers have to trust their knowledge and determine if the information is accurate, objective, and supported by appropriate references and links.
- Use of a tool can make systematic evaluation of websites consistant, particularly when these resources are needed as information support in a perioperative nursing project.

At many workplaces there is one person known for sharing interesting bits of information by forwarding e-mails or bringing in newspaper and Internet articles. While cartoons and jokes may be amusing, sometimes the information is composed of doubtful facts, including terrible crime threats, political scandals, and unusual medical treatments. The same stories that might have been kindly dismissed when discussed in the break room are somehow thought to be more substantial and reliable because they are in print. Casually judging the value of these stories is easy when the outcome is unimportant. The evaluation of information is more difficult when the outcome is more significant, such as when when people's health or lives are involved. The provision of good health care should be supported by current, reliable, and authoritative information. Evaluating sources is an important health care skill.

Words on paper or on a webpage are just data if no one reads the material. Data has little value until it is understood and used by an individual. Data becomes

The author has nothing to disclose.
Science and Engineering Library, University of Texas at Arlington, PO Box 19497, B03 Nedderman Hall, 416 Yates Street, Arlington, TX 76019, USA
E-mail address: hough@uta.edu

information only when a person has read and understood its potential significance. Knowledge is the ability to recall and use information as input into decisions.[1] Nurses may become aware of volumes of information as more people use the Internet for communication. A mere 150 years ago, the only reliable way to communicate across large distances was by the written word. While technology may have changed the speed, form, and volume of information being transferred, people are not significantly different. We still need reliable information to solve physical and social problems. The assessment of information provided by others has always been based on the context of social structures and values.

SOCIAL CONSTRAINTS OF INFORMATION

The concept of the suitability of information is based in its utility. By definition, data does not become information unless it is understood by the user.[2] Language and tone affect emotional responses to information, and emotions affect comprehension. Relevancy is also a component of suitability. Informed decisions can only be made when the information is relevant to the issue at hand. User expectations, the match between available data and what is needed, timeliness, and the focus of the information affect relevancy.[3] An information user is better able to judge the suitability of sources if the original question or need is understood.

The concept of authority in information is part of a social structure. Patients and colleagues look to nurses and other health care providers as knowledgeable information providers, valuing the expertise of these professionals. Expertise is assessed through awareness of length of practice, professional credentials, place of employment, relevancy of the expert's prior work, and recognition by other professionals.

The methods of evaluating printed materials can be compared to judging the value of information transmitted orally. For example, more questions may arise regarding the reliability of health care research information relayed by a teenage supermarket cashier than there would be if the same materials are discussed in a professional seminar by a scientist on the research team. Personnel facts transmitted by the chief executive officer of the hospital may be assessed as more valuable than those told by a neighbor employed in a different profession. The first example is one of authority and the second, of relevancy. Resources in print or from the Internet can be assessed in a similar manner. Most reliable documents can be obtained from recognized organizations' websites or can be checked for authors' names, credentials, and affiliations. Responsible journals and books are published by known and respected publishers. A wise person considers how any information is obtained and judges its value based on similar criteria regardless of format.

CRITERIA FOR ASSESSING INFORMATION SOURCES

Understand the need for the information. It is important to appreciate the variables that need to be addressed by this information and the impact of the information itself. A document, video, or other resource may not be relevant if the amount or language of the information inappropriate. The coverage may be too broad or narrow. The language may be too scholarly or elementary. When examining a document for suitability, consider when it was created and its intended audience. Authors write with specific audiences in mind, and material is less relevant if the document content and the audience do not correspond. An example of audience mismatch may be standard educational materials written at a high school level being provided to a patient requiring low-literacy information. Attitudes and health care knowledge also change, and it is important to be aware of when materials were originally produced.

After the need and use of the information is understood, the materials themselves can be assessed. Authority, objectivity, documentation, and verifiability are common assessment variables. Some of the most important aspects of reliability are relatively simple to assess. If there are multiple spelling and grammar errors, the content may have additional problems in the accuracy of facts or other content. If there is no indication of how to contact the author or website for clarification, these errors cannot be challenged or corrected. Responsible authors take care in how their work is presented. They also provide a means of contact for feedback and corrections. An example of suspect reliability is *Wikipedia*; the contributors remain anonymous and do not have to provide contact information to the organization. Anonymous sources like *Wikipedia* entries can be used as a beginning discovery tool for basic terms and concepts but should not be considered authoritative.

Authority usually is judged by determining if the author or organization that produced the material is reliable. Scholarly resources are written by those with appropriate academic credentials. Sometimes an author is not specified. In these cases, an organization or agency accepts responsibility for the content. Sponsorship from a reputable organization or being posted on the organization's website carries weight similar to an article published in a respected journal. Articles from the *American Cancer Society* website or published in the *AORN Journal*, by the Association of Operating Room Nurses, should be considered more reliable than a local news organization. Government agencies should also be considered more reliable than many other sources. If a news story is reporting about research published elsewhere, consider using the original source, not the news report. When the reliability of the responsible agent is unknown, other documents from a respected source or website may provide evidence of reliability.

Objectivity and considerations regarding bias may occasionally be a subjective assessment depending on the kind of information needed. The sense of objectivity is often gathered from the tone of language and the belief that the authors of a document are trying to present a balanced discussion of a topic. However, the reader's values, attitudes, feelings, or beliefs affect this perception. An example of different appreciations of objectivity may be observed from reactions to any one of a number of controversial issues. Any given report may be viewed by the reader as biased if it does not provide some level of support for the reader's views. Objectivity is supported in reports of scientific studies when the applicability and usefulness of the research is discussed. Resources produced by companies intending to sell goods or services are often seen as biased but may be useful. Lowered objectivity and higher acceptability of bias may be appropriate if relevancy is high.

Supportive documentation in the form of references, links, and other means for the reader to learn more about the topic helps to authenticate the information being presented. References included in a research report should be of at least the same scholarly level as the report. Internet sources should provide links to other resources on the general topic. Reliability is increased if the references and links are associated with other scholars' works or respected organizations' materials. In some cases there are only a few highly qualified experts in a field, and references to those experts should be expected.

EVALUATION TOOLS

Websites can be reviewed just like movies and books. Professional journals and organizations will often recommend specific resources. Some information users have found that developing and using a simple checklist tool to maintain a consistent quality of source materials is helpful. An individual can create a personal tool to

Date assessed: 1/5/2012				**TOTAL SCORE**: 50/52		
				(Excellent)		
Webpage title/URL: *AORN, Free Online Education*; http://www.aorn.org/FreeCE/						
Assessment purpose: Access to free perioperative nursing CEUs for Jones Hospital Nurses (Hospital Goal 1.2.1)						
Scoring: (0) very poor, (1) poor, (2) fair, (3) good, (4) excellent;						
Total scores: 0-6 very poor, 7-20, poor, 21-32 fair, 32-45 good, 46-52 excellent						

Relevancy						
	Very Poor	Poor	Fair	Good	Excellent	Totals
Audience clearly identified on resource				3		
Audience match to purpose					4	
Appropriate language for audience					4	
Coverage relative to purpose					4	
Timeliness relative to purpose					4	
Relevancy: Total Possible 20				3	16	**19**

Reliability						
	Very Poor	Poor	Fair	Good	Excellent	Totals
Author name & credentials included				3		
Reliable website/organization/publisher					4	
Contact information included					4	
Date created/updated included/published					4	
Spelling & grammar correct					4	
Information appears accurate					4	
Objective report/ bias acceptable					4	
Appropriate references, links					4	
Reliability: Total Possible 32				3	28	**31**

Comments:	Assuming nursing CEUs - AORN site					
	Responsible agency assumed from heading & copyright information					
	Explicit references not necessary at this level; Links work					
	Membership required for some units					
Name of Assessor: Mary Smith	*Review dates*					

Fig. 1. Example tool.

systematically evaluate resources. The assessment tool can then be used to compare the quality of a variety of resources (**Fig. 1**).

The two major categories of a valid assessment are relevancy and reliability.[4] For webpage assessment, components of relevancy are audience, coverage, timeliness, and language. Components of reliability are accuracy, authority, currency, sponsorship, objectivity, and authentication. An evaluation tool may include these terms as checklist reminders. Assessment can be quantitative or qualitative; a qualitative scale might have related values including *not at all, somewhat, reasonable, good,* and *excellent.* An overall assessment would lean toward one value or another. A quantitative assessment of meeting the criteria can be the use of these terms in the form of a 5-point Likert scale, where a value is assigned to each of the points. In the case of quantitative scale, an assigned minimal total score would determine the overall accessibility of the resource. Since each resource is assessed separately relative to meeting some general or specific need, there would need to be one copy of the tool for each resource. An appropriate reference to the resource, usually title and retrieval information, date of assessment, and purpose of assessment, should also be included.

The use of an evaluation tool ensures that the same elements are examined consistently. Scanning webpages can be very tiring, and opinions can change based on this fatigue. The personal interests of the evaluator can also alter perceptions of relevancy. Documenting the reason for the evaluation reminds the evaluator of the specific need and required relevancy, as shown in the example in **Fig. 1**, which shows the focus on perioperative nursing continuing education hours (CE) as opposed to any other specialization. A quantitative assessment, also includes the evaluation points associated with website relevancy and reliability assessments (see **Fig. 1**). A CE website for a perioperative nurse would have to be current (*timeliness*) and for nurses (*audience*). A reliable website that the nurse could use and would use more than once, ideally, should be kept up to date by a recognized, respected organization (*author*, *reliable*). To ensure that the website is actually from that organization and not from an unethical entity engaged in a criminal act like information theft, it is important that there be contact information for the organization. Good spelling, grammar, references, and links are significant clues because a respected organization would present itself well and respect the audience. Above all, the assessor has to trust his or her knowledge that the site as a whole makes sense, particularly in terms of information accuracy and bias potential. The consistent reminder to look for these elements ensures that quality resources will be identified because, for example, a good web page can be compared with any other good web page even if the web pages differ in the reasons why they obtained that assessment. Consistency can be even more important when a project extends over long periods of time or when more than one person is involved. If a list of resources is going to be maintained over time, adding dates to reviews is also valuable because organizations change their websites, and universal resource locations (URL) disappear.

SUMMARY

Several variables should be considered when assessing information sources. Many of these variables are understood and used in interpersonal situations or when using print sources. Assessment of Internet resources has not always been approached in the same manner, but the concepts are transferable. Understanding what information is applicable, who created the source, who or what supports its continuation as a resource, how it can be authenticated, and how it will be used are all critical aspects reliability. The information user's knowledge, combined with systematic consideration of these variables, is needed to ensure the necessary information is gathered and used appropriately. An evaluation tool can be very useful for maintaining assessment consistency over time.[1]

REFERENCES

1. Rowley J, Hartley R. Organizing knowledge: an introduction to managing access to information. Ashgate Publishing, Ltd; 2006.
2. Ackoff RL. From data to wisdom. J Appl Sys Anal 1989;16:3–9.
3. Wallace DP. Knowledge management: historical and cross-disciplinary themes. Westport (CT): Libraries Unlimited; 2007.
4. Burns N, Grove SK, Gray J. Understanding nursing research: building an evidence-based practice. 5th edition. Maryland Heights (MO): Elsevier/Saunders; 2011.

Maintaining Nursing Knowledge Using Bibliographic Management Software

Eileen Stec, MS, MSW

KEYWORDS

- Bibliographic management • Citation management • Journal citations
- Evidence-based practice • Continuing nursing education

KEY POINTS

- To engage in evidence-based practice, perioperative nurses should be regularly accessing literature on pertinent practice subjects.
- Use of bibliographic management software can help nurses sift through databases to find literature content that meets their needs.

Two bibliographic management products are compared in this article, RefWorks 2.0, produced by ProQuest LLC and EndNote v.X5, produced by Thomson Reuters. For the purposes of the product comparison the EndNote, a stand-alone client was loaded on an individual computer and the RefWorks Web-based, institutional version was used. Both applications were tested on the Microsoft XP Operating System using the Internet Explorer Web browser. The databases used for searching are the free PubMed database and the subscription-based Cumulative Index for Nursing and Allied Health Literature (CINAHL) database.

The features of the two applications selected for comparison were based on an assumption that professional perioperative nurses will be using the software to remain current in their field. Neither features used to generate bibliographies for publication nor inserting footnotes into papers will be assessed. Several other no-cost bibliographic management software applications exist including Zotero, Mendeley, BibTex, and citulike. These applications will not be reviewed in this article. Ovadia[1] provides information regarding the aforementioned no-cost bibliographic management products and their respective features.

The author has nothing to disclose.
Mabel Smith Douglass Library, Rutgers, The State University of New Jersey, 8 Chapel Drive, New Brunswick, NJ 08901, USA
E-mail address: estec@rci.rutgers.edu

Perioperative Nursing Clinics 7 (2012) 195–200
doi:10.1016/j.cpen.2012.02.004
1556-7931/12/$ – see front matter © 2012 Elsevier Inc. All rights reserved.

ENDNOTE

EndNote software allows storage of portable document format (.pdf) journal articles. The stored .pdf full-text articles may be highlighted and annotated. The digital tools included serve the same purpose as a highlighting marker to color portions of printed text or a sticky-note allowing the nurse to return quickly to important information and personal comments she or he made concerning portions of the article. All the citation fields—including but not limited to—keywords, author, and abstracts associated with a citation can be edited and searched after storage.

Searching PubMed from Within the EndNote Product

Some users prefer the ease of searching the PubMed database from within the bibliographic program. Searching from within bibliographic management software can severely limit the citation results a nurse retrieves. Patient care can be compromised when poor search technique results in omission of important journal articles. Some search options and hints can be seen and utilized only when searching the native PubMed index. For example, when keying in a search term or phrase in PubMed a drop-down box opens offering suggested vocabulary for the search.

Using the search query *pain management* AND *best practice* AND *perioperative* in PubMed as text terms yielded the highest, most relevant results. Searching the same phrases as Medical Subject Headings (MeSH) yielded no results. Unless the perioperative nurse knows MeSH vocabulary, this search approach should be avoided because it may otherwise yield no results.

Searching PubMed Without Using EndNote Software and Importing the Results

While searching PubMed directly from the PubMed Web site, suggested phrases could be seen when a term is keyed in and a suggested term or phrase can be selected from a drop-down menu beneath the search box (**Fig. 1**). For example, *pain management nursing* was a suggestion offered when *pain management* was keyed into the search box. Also, *best practices* was additionally offered rather than just the singular form *best practice*. The suggested search phrases were only offered when one search phrase was keyed into the search box at a time. Combining search terms or phrases with AND, OR, or NOT within the same search line disables the suggestion search terms. Consequently, each phrase was searched separately for this article. By using the advanced search feature, individual searches saved in the history box allow the searcher to combine the result sets in the history. PubMed tutorials may be accessed on the Internet.[2]

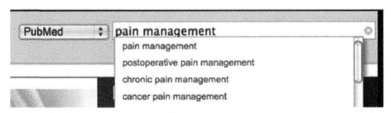

Fig. 1. PubMed *pain management* search.

Searching CINAHL

Connecting directly from an institutional subscription of the CINAHL index to the computer where EndNote was loaded could not be accomplished. Therefore, searching CINAHL within EndNote was not tested. Email from EndNote tech support indicated that if a nurse has an individual subscription, export directly into EndNote from CINAHL could be possible. Exporting citations from within CINAHL to a stand-alone version of EndNote was accomplished quickly.

Attaching or Accessing Full Text of an Article

The Ebscohost version of CINAHL offers a feature to export to EndNote Web allowing uploading citations to a personal account (free for the first 2 years) along with the full text of any article citations available in the .pdf file format. The .pdf files may also be attached manually in EndNote stand-alone version to a citation after first downloading an individual journal article to the computer. Attaching the article to the citation helps avoid the clutter and potential loss of printed journal articles.

Help/Tutorials

Getting started training tutorials provided for EndNote are informative and broken into modules. The learning curve is moderately steep for a novice, as it would be for any powerful application. The tutorials may be freely accessed online.[3] Individual assistance requested via email from EndNote did not prove adequate to connect to an institutional CINAHL subscription.

Cost

The EndNote cost is moderate, particularly if purchased with an academic discount. Information regarding academic discount pricing is available only through your educational institution or visiting the Thomson Reuters purchase page for information regarding "academic solutions." Expect to spend $200 to $300; you then own the software permanently. The purchase price includes a free 2-year Web account allowing collections to be saved for access via the Internet. A perioperative nurse would need more than a single copy of EndNote to access the personal Web collections from different computers. This begs the question, "Why make a Web accessible collection at all?" Perhaps the best and only reason to create a Web collection in EndNote would be to safeguard citations in the event of a catastrophic computer event, such as a failure of a hard drive (**Table 1**).

REFWORKS

A notable feature and requirement when using Refworks is that it is accessible from any Internet accessible computer via a Web browser. After creating a search in PubMed a perioperative nurse can save the search as a Really Simple Syndication (RSS) feed. The RSS feature as described in the RefWorks help files[4] allows the nurse to run the same search on a regular basis retrieving any new literature fitting the criteria of the saved search. The National Library of Medicine (NLM)[5] loads new citations into PubMed Tuesday through Friday, allowing the nursing professional to check for the most recent articles by running the RSS feed feature on a regular basis. Weekly or monthly updates should be sufficient for most needs; daily uploads by the NLM does not automatically yield new article citations. The updates occur as publishers release citation files to the NLM. NLM uploads any citations supplied by a publisher. If journal articles relating to your specific topic are not being published, no new articles will be available.

Table 1 Bibliographic management software comparison		
	EndNote	**RefWorks**
Searching PubMed	Both products successfully searched PubMed from within the product itself. Neither product provided the richness of search assistance the PubMed site provided for itself.	
Searching CINAHL	Neither product could access CINAHL through the product itself.	
Cost	One-time product cost between $200 and $300 to the nurse, depending on availability of academic discount.	Institutional subscription free to nurses of the institution. Individual subscriptions available for $100 per year.
Tutorials and Help features	Internet tutorials available for free. Email support was quick but not useful.	Internet tutorials available for free. Information to import PubMed results files is incorrect.
Other features	Can attach journal article files to citations, highlight, and include personal comments on articles.	Institutional subscriptions allow attachment of journal article files.
Issues	Search results can be stored on either the nurse's computer or on the Internet (free for first 2 years).	Search results must be stored on the Internet.

Searching via RefWorks Versus a Search from the Database and Ingesting Citations into RefWorks

Creating a personal account and login is the first step. In the case of an institutional subscription, there is no individual cost to the nurse. RefWorks also automatically creates storage for search results on the Web with the creation of a personal account. Personal subscriptions are paid for annually by the subscriber and may be renewed without loss of stored citations.

Searching PubMed from within RefWorks provides quick search or advanced search options, allowing either individual or all fields search. As with the PubMed search discussed earlier for EndNote, practitioners are advised to try a search concept directly within PubMed first to ascertain the most appropriate search terms or concepts available.

Importing references from PubMed is multi-stepped and should be approached with caution. Be certain when working in PubMed all the search results you wish to import are displayed on one browser page. If you decide to display only 20 results per page but would like to import all 28 results, the last 8 citations will be lost. The Help feature of RefWorks provides steps for import, including using the Web browser's "save as" function. These directions did not work as described in the RefWorks help materials. It was necessary to follow the import directions to display the search results, ignoring the "save as" steps. Copying the properly formatted display from the Web browser, then using the "import from text" option, THEN copying and pasting the results directly into the area provided was the only successful method to export citations from PubMed and import into RefWorks. If an institutional subscription to Medline is available, it is preferable to search within Medline for export of citations rather than using PubMed.

Other Features

Attachment of a full text article to a citation is possible when a citation is being edited or added manually under only one circumstance. The attachment feature is available for organization-wide subscriptions only. Individual subscribers cannot attach a full-text article to a citation.

Perioperative nurses with access to RefWorks via the same institutional subscription may share citations. Shared access allows one storage point for joint projects or journal discussion groups. Unfortunately, nurses with RefWorks access from different institutions may not share a central storage space.

Tutorials and Cost

RefWorks tutorials are available online.[6] Tutorials are broken into short—2- to 4-minute—segments. The size of the RefWorks tutorials is preferable to EndNote's longer tutorials for return users; a casual user may return to relearn only the features she needs versus repeating EndNotes' multi-feature tutorials. Conversely, EndNote tutorials may describe several tools or features in a tutorial providing an overview of the process as well as instruction. The cost for an institutional subscription is borne by the institution, not the individual. As with any institutional subscription, cost is negotiated and varies. Individuals may subscribe for $100 annually. Software is accessed only online and updated versions of RefWorks are available immediately and automatically. This can be disconcerting to the unsuspecting—suddenly viewing new features or interface changes. However, there is no additional fee for new versions. Individual subscriptions must be renewed annually for continued access to the software citations saved at RefWorks' online site.

SUMMARY

Both EndNote and RefWorks are produced by reputable companies that have been in existence for some time, ProQuest and Thomson Reuters, respectively. This is a good thing to know if one is spending money for software—the company can be expected to continue to provide customer support and upgrades. Both EndNote and RefWorks are good products albeit not perfect. The deciding factor for the perioperative nurse may very well come down to availability and cost. If the nurse's institution has subscribed to RefWorks, the software is available to him or her at no cost. If an institutional subscription to RefWorks is not available, the next feature for consideration after cost should be the appropriateness of the product and the intended use. EndNote is fine for one nurse who always uses the same computer for his or her scholarly journal research. Used for several years, EndNote will be less expensive than RefWorks, but results may be kept on an individual computer without cost only after the initial 2 years of free Internet storage. RefWorks, on the other hand is most useful to the nurse who needs access from more than one Internet-connected computer. The other features and limitations between the two products come down to the value the individual perioperative nurse places on tutorials and help-desk service, storing full-text documents with citations, and the ability to share the citations with other nurses. The last feature will not be available to independent practitioners regardless of the product.

REFERENCES

1. Ovadia S. Managing citations with cost-free tools. Behav Soc Sci Librarian 2011;30: 107–11.

2. PubMed. PubMed tutorials. Available at: http://www.nlm.nih.gov/bsd/disted/pubmedtutorial/index.html. Accessed January 13, 2012.
3. Endnote. Endnote tutorials. Available at: http://endnote.com/training/. Accessed January 13, 2012.
4. Refworks. RefWorks help file. Available at: http://www.refworks.com.proxy.libraries.rutgers.edu/refworks2/help/RefWorks2.htm. Accessed January 13, 2012.
5. U.S. National Library of Medicine: National Institutes of Health. Available at: http://www.nlm.nih.gov/. Accessed January 13, 2012.
6. RefWorks 2.0 Fundamentals tutorial. Available at: http://www.refworks-cos.com/refworks/tutorials/basic.html. Accessed January 13, 2012.

Copyright and the Perioperative Nurse

Helen Hough, MLS, BS, BA[a],*, Kristen Priddy, RNC-Ob, MSN, CNS[b]

KEYWORDS

- Copyright • Internet • Writing for publication • Teaching materials • Liability

KEY POINTS

- The authors or creators of products including written works, graphics, photographs, and digital objects have rights to determine how these products can be used.
- Permission to use the products of other people's creative endeavors should be obtained.
- Use of these products without permission can result in fines.
- There are several methods of protection against copyright liability.

Every time a perioperative nurse gives a patient printed instructions to take home, that nurse is involved with issues related to copyright. When a person makes photocopies to share with others, downloads a file or graphic to use at work, provides handouts at an in-service or a class, or writes for publication, the person is involved with copyright regulations. A basic understanding of why copyright exists, what it involves, and how it impacts the health care provider is important. Knowledge of the opportunities related to copyright fair use allows some flexibility. Failure to abide by copyright regulations can financially impact both the provider and the institution where the provider works. Using this knowledge can protect the nurse from lawsuits.

Stories are often heard about downloading online songs and movies and how easy this is to do. In addition, stories are related about how music or film companies try to prevent these downloads. The person who is trying to obtain useful resources may not appreciate why there is restricted access on some publications by the publisher

The authors have nothing to disclose.

Authors' Legal Statement: We are information and nurse professionals, not lawyers. This intellectual property information is provided for general purposes only. If you believe you have a legal concern, please contact a licensed legal professional. If you are associated with a government agency or corporation, also consider contacting your business's legal representation.

[a] Science and Engineering Library, University of Texas at Arlington, PO Box 19497, B03 Nedderman Hall, 416 Yeats Street, Arlington, TX 76019, USA

[b] College of Nursing, The University of Texas at Arlington, Box 19407, 622 Pickard Hall, 411 South Nedderman Drive, Arlington, TX 76019, USA

* Corresponding author.

E-mail address: hough@uta.edu

Perioperative Nursing Clinics 7 (2012) 201–210

doi:10.1016/j.cpen.2012.02.008

or owner when these things can be easy to see and copy from another venue. After all, how could these alternate copies affect these companies? Besides, with a slight bit of technical skill, downloading files or photocopying articles or books is often easy to do. What most people do not realize is that these actions may be in violation of the US Copyright Act[1] and, depending on the circumstances, people and the companies they work for may be liable for inappropriate reproduction and distribution of materials owned by others.

As an exercise for understanding copyright, consider a car as a metaphor for a book, graphic, or song. A person can buy one or more cars or can buy one or more copies of a book or similar resource. That person owns those specific objects, not all copies of that object. The key to a specific car does not open all cars of the make and model. If a person attempts to manufacture more of those cars and sell them without permission from the original manufacturer, the lawyers at the company holding the right to manufacture those cars will probably seek financial reparations. The person who wants more of the cars has a few options including (a) buying, (b) formally borrowing, or (c) renting them from the manufacturer or dealer. The person could alternatively choose to buy similar cars from other manufacturers or build really nice, even better, new cars. Intellectual property in the form of words, music, and graphics is just as much property as are physical objects like cars. The ownership of a specific make and model of a car does not give a person the right to manufacture more of those cars, just as owning a book or painting does not give the right to that owner to make copies of that book or painting and distribute those copies. The person who has obtained one car or one copy of a book, painting, or other creative work has exactly that, one item. A person can own a car, text, or picture and keep, loan, rent, or sell that specific car, text, or picture, but not other copies of that product.

Ownership options fall within the copyright, trademark, or patent laws when an item is the result of intellectual property such as a person's ideas. Patents are related to inventions, and trademarks are related to images or text that represent an entity including a company or product. Copyright law is related to the ownership of text, music, presentations, and images fixed in tangible form. These forms include the physical object itself, print copies, or digital formats. Through the intellectual property laws, people own the products of their ideas and creations and have the right to determine how these products are made available to others.

THE US CONSTITUTION

In the United States, copyright is based on the US Constitution. It is not just within the Bill of Rights or the Amendments, but within the Constitution itself. Article 1[2] defines the power of the US Congress. Section 8, Clause 8 of Article 1 states that Congress has the power "To promote the Progress of Science and useful Arts, by securing for limited Times to Authors and Inventors the exclusive Right to their respective Writings and Discoveries."[2] From this statement comes the American intellectual property laws that Congress has passed, including the Digital Millennium Copyright Act.[3] Over the past 2 centuries these laws have changed to reflect American social concerns and technological developments. Many other countries currently have similar laws, some more restrictive and others less restrictive than American laws. Of course, current technology enables the transmission of intellectual property, the tangible record of ideas, across international borders. It can be difficult to determine who created what and where it was created. However, the information about the ownership of things recorded as electronic files, printed resources, and images including pictures can also be transmitted across borders. The United States has treaties with many countries, and people who violate intellectual property laws can face legal problems in other countries.

Cultural variations in the values placed on ideas further complicate issues relating to intellectual property laws. In some cultures, the concept that a person or corporation can truly own the products of an idea is incomprehensible; good ideas are to be used to benefit members of the larger community. Even if the concept of the ownership of ideas is part of a person's worldview, there is often a lack of understanding of the difference between owning an object created as a result of that idea and having the right to distribute copies of that object. When tangible objects are a product of an idea, these products can be owned and controlled by the author or creator. A common result of the failure to understand both of these views, ownership of an idea or the objects that are created from them, is that there are many incidences of *intellectual property theft*. An example of intellectual theft often comes in the form of counterfeiting. Counterfeiting is defined as systematic copying of an image, object, product, or computer file without paying for it and the selling these copies as the original or a legitimate, registered, and faithful reproduction of the original concept.[4] Sometimes the illegal copy is not as reliable as the appropriately manufactured product, as has been shown in counterfeit drugs. Sometimes the copy is perfectly acceptable but the owner/creator or copyright holder is not compensated for the skill and effort that went into the creation of the object; a book, painting, photograph, piece of art, computer program, or other material.

Another interesting analogy to paying for intellectual property is paying for health care. People who create things by writing, creating graphics, developing programs, and so on, learned how to do these activities. They spent time and money developing these skills, often over years. They usually earn their living by producing these resources. If creative work was easy, anyone could create high quality materials. The provision of high quality nursing care has similar features. Perioperative nurses and other health care providers spend years learning and developing the skills to provide valuable care. On the other hand, this care is expensive and many consumers do not want to pay the high costs related to this care. Just as nurses and other providers deserve reasonable compensation for their labors, authors and artists should be paid for theirs. Using resources without fairly compensating their creators does not respect the time, education, intellectual effort, or other costs associated with the resources. Only if the products of this time and labor are freely given should others feel free to take them.

COPYRIGHT

Copyrights are the rights provided to creators that allow them control regarding the use of their products of their intellectual efforts. These rights and privileges include the right to reproduce the work. Another right is the right to distribute the work, including creating print copies and distribution over the Internet or by other methods, including digital versions. An author or creator can also determine who can publicly perform certain types of works and where these performances are permitted, including publicly playing recordings. Permissions for use of materials still under copyright protection include the right to restrict public presentation of recordings. Only the author or creator has the right to allow others some or all of these privileges (**Table 1**). The author or creator can sell some or all of these privileges to others. These rights are usually transferred by contract, just like one would transfer ownership or allow the renting of a car. Both the creator and the recipient should keep copies of these contracts.

Table 1	
Copyright owner rights	
Right	Example
Reproduce	Make a copy
Create derivative work	Use a work as basis for new work
Distribute work	Electronically distribute/publish copies
Publicly perform work	Publicly perform
Publicly play recording	Publicly play recordings
Publicly display work	Publicly display image on computer screen
Allow/contract others these rights	Permission to use, perform, or distribute

AMERICAN COPYRIGHTABLE INTELLECTUAL PROPERTY

American intellectual property includes traditional written products like text, plays, and musical scores. Artistic products including graphics, photos, and images are also intellectual property. Performances and recordings of these performances as well as other works including tests, assessment instruments, and computer programs are protected. Materials that are copyrighted are those works fixed in tangible form, meaning that the idea has been written, drawn, photographed, or otherwise recorded in any one of a variety of media including print and digital formats. A person can see or touch the object that is the result of the development of the idea. These products are copyrighted. Some ideas, processes, methods, and systems described in standard copyrighted works are not considered copyrighted.

Some things are not considered original creative works, including facts and works composed of these facts. Included also in the class of nonoriginal works are logical, comprehensive compilations like phone books. Other resources were never eligible for copyright protection, and others have passed the duration of protection in effect at the creation or registration of the resource or renewal of these rights. US federal government publications are not eligible for coverage because these are created with public funds; they are automatically within the public domain. Government agencies may use some materials with permission of the creators and without compromising the owners' reproduction rights; examples of this use can include the A.D.A.M. graphics, which are often used in MedlinePlus Web pages.[5] A.D.A.M. Inc has retained the right to sell these graphics even though the graphics are used in government publications. State and local government agency resources are copyright protected because they are not federal documents.

Copyright privileges exist for limited periods, as indicated in the US Constitution.[1] Materials are in the public domain when copyright protections do not exist for the author or creator of that object. Some products have never been protected, including most federal government publications, whereas other products lapse into the public domain after specific periods. These periods are governed by the copyright laws in existence at the time of the creation or registration of the resource, by renewal of these rights by the owners, or as otherwise indicated by law.

Owners or creators can also choose to expressly donate their creative works to the public. An example of these donated creative works is freeware, which the author has chosen to make available without restriction. Other limited donated works may be identified by Creative Commons (CC) licensure or other open access initiatives.[6,7] CC[6] is a nonprofit organization that advocates and supports legal and technical methods that increase creativity and sharing of digital resources. One of these methods is the CC copyright license. The CC licenses have a structure that allows the creator/author of digital works to clearly specify how these works may be used by others including copying, distribution, editing, and remixing. Open access is an international movement among scholars and researchers to provide quality research materials at low or no cost to the reader. An example of one of the leading organizations in this movement is the Scholarly Publishing and Academic Resources Coalition (SPARC).[7] Many colleges, universities, and research institutions have institutional repositories where members of the organization can deposit copies of their works so the public can access them.

Scholars may be required to sign over their copyrights to publishers as a part of the publication process. Often authors sign contracts without realizing the contract allows the publisher to become the copyright holder and the author no longer has any rights to the creative work. Contracts between author and publisher may be modified by the participants of the contract. A common modification is the SPARC author addendum, which includes reserving the right to keep a copy of the work in the author's institutional repository.[8] The author addendum can also allow the author to use these works in classes he or she teaches. Licensed legal experts in copyright law are best able to interpret what materials might be copyrighted, what cannot be protected, and which materials are no longer protected.

LEGAL CONSEQUENCES

Individuals and companies may make significant money on copyrighted materials. At the very least, there are authors, illustrators, programmers, and people in publishing, music, and movie industries who make their living as a result of creative efforts. Copyright infringement, like stealing cars, can have expensive repercussions. If a charge of willful copyright infringement is shown true in an American court, currently a fine of up to $150,000 for each act can be rendered in addition to attorneys' fees and other legal costs. Willful infringement means the person knew about copyright and violated it anyway. Unintentional infringement is usually limited to damage (loss of income) as well as the attorneys' and other legal fees. Either intentional or unintentional infringement can result in significant costs to the person who violated these laws. As in the case of malpractice suits, social and emotional costs are high even if the defendant is found innocent.

WHAT IS COPYRIGHT PROTECTED?

US copyright applies to United States materials and those created or registered in countries with which the United States has treaties.[1] As of 2011, materials published prior to 1923 are in public domain and may be used freely (**Table 2**). Materials published between 1923 and 1963 that are marked with the copyright symbol are in the public domain if the copyrights have not been renewed. Materials published between these two dates and formally renewed are still protected. The oldest currently copyrighted materials will go into public domain in 2019 unless Congress changes the law and extends these rights. An extension was granted to materials published between 1964 and 1978 because Congress extended copyright protection periods. Materials published between 1964 and 1978 were eligible for automatic renewal and are still under copyright.

Materials created after 1978, whether formally published or not, are copyright protected for the life of the author/creator plus 70 years. In other words, it does not matter if a book, painting, photograph, graphic, computer program, audio recording, video recording, or personal diary is old by someone's definition of old. Old enough is defined

Table 2		
Copyright protection time period		
Published	**Copyright Length**	**Public Domain**
Before 1923	Now in public domain	Yes
1923–1963, not renewed[a]	28 y, with ©	Maybe
1923–1978, renewed[a]	95 y, with ©	No
After 1978	Life of author/creator + 70 y	No
Never published	Life of author/creator + 70 y	No

[a] Check Stanford "Determinator" for renewal status.

Modified from Harper GK. Fair use of copyrighted materials Copyright Crash Course. Published 2007. Available at: http://copyright.lib.utexas.edu/copypol2.html. Accessed March 13, 2012.

by current copyright law. It does not matter if these objects have copyright symbols on them or not. The symbol is not currently required. Many things can still be under copyright. If materials have been created within the past 30 years, simply the act of creating them entitles the authors/creators the copyright privileges associated with those products.

EDUCATIONAL/FAIR USE

There is a little flexibility in the copyright law for commentary about intellectual property as well as educational and research use of these products. Most of this flexibility, called *fair use*, is based in physical in-class use, student use, individual use, and use within limited collaborative research venues. Online courses are more restricted because of the course distribution method. Posting products on the Internet can cause multiple copies to be easily created and accessed. Without care by the person posting the document, image, or file, an Internet environment can unintentionally allow people from around the world access to the protected material. This lack of care can result in the person posting the item being at risk for either intentional or unintentional copyright infringement, depending on the circumstances. People are not legally authorized to copy and post text or graphics on the Internet, even if this posting is for a class of patients, a class of students, or for some other worthy purpose. The TEACH Act clarifies and provides additional limitations related to copyright for online course work.[9]

FAIR USE FOUR FACTORS

Interpretation of fair use as it relates to copyright can be complicated. The current United States copyright laws are old enough to be nonspecific relative to technological advances, and the courts have not provided consistent interpretations. Some courts have favored educational use, and others have leaned toward favoring the copyright owner, particularly when the owner is a company or corporation that has suffered economic damage from copyright infringement.

Generally, there are four factors (**Table 3**) weighing in on fair use, all of which are related to money.[10] These factors are the (a) character of the use, (b) nature of the work, (c) percentage of the work being used, and (d) marketability of the material. The character of the use is associated with how materials are being used.

Character of use is judged in the context of material being used in a nonprofit, educational, or personal setting (**Box 1**). A consideration, even in a nonprofit or educational setting, is that people may be earning money as a result of this use. Even

Table 3
Four factors of fair use

Factor	Likely Fair Use	Likely Infringement
Character of use	Nonprofit, educational, personal	Commercial [$$]
Nature of work?	Fact, published	Imaginative, unpublished [→ new/creative, $]
Amount used	Small amount (<10%)	A lot (>15%) [→ reproduction]
Effect on original's marketability	Password/time protection	Market competition; action done to avoid fees

in a nonprofit or educational setting, doctors, nurses, health care providers, teachers, and many others are getting paid and therefore misusing copyrightable materials, resulting in earnings from someone else's idea and labor.

The second factor, the **nature of the work** or material, is that a fact, set of facts, or materials already published may be easily available. Weighing against ease of access is that some materials are the result of creative endeavors that cannot be produced by just anyone. The material may be unpublished and the author/creator may be able to earn some income as a result of documenting these ideas.

The **amount of copyright** materials used is also considered. A small amount, usually less than 10% of the entire work, is often considered negligible. This negligible amount is not usually a problem. More than 15% of an entire work, or in the case of something like a book or a movie, the disclosure of full plot line or conclusion might be considered infringement. A consideration with objects like graphics is that whereas the object itself may be small, it is the percentage of use of that object that is evaluated, not the size of the object. One cannot copy and use an entire graphic because the entire graphic is the entire work.

Often the most significant factor is the effect on the **marketability of the material**. There may be less liability in a court of law for the person or corporation distributing copyrighted materials without permission if access to material is controlled by password and/or time constraints. Most courts will probably not look favorably at a person or company engaging in the distribution of copyrighted materials, even in restricted environments, if the intention of the distribution is to avoid paying fees for the use of the material.

PLAGIARISM

Plagiarism is related to but may not constitute copyright infringement. Plagiarism may be considered fraud. If a person presents prior work or knowledge from someone else's work as new or one's own, this representation is not truthful. If the person is

Box 1
Copyrighted materials

- Creative efforts fixed in tangible forms including text, images, and digital formats
- Potentially income-generating
- Constitutionally based rights

presenting this work for academic credit, monetary reward, or purposes of prestige, the person is misrepresenting his or her abilities. In academic and scientific environments such as hospitals, this presentation is called plagiarism. Even self-plagiarism can occur if older work is submitted as new. The author/creator may own the work, and it is the misrepresentation of the materials that is the problem. When discussing previously published or submitted materials, the author or creator should document these facts in any new materials.

LIKELIHOOD OF BEING CAUGHT

Cases of copyright violation have not been that common in courts of law. Most court cases are expensive, and violations are commonly settled out of court. The copyright holder may ask the person engaging in violation of the holder's right to stop distributing materials however the distribution is determined. Often the violator will stop. Cases are brought to court when the risk of losing income outweighs the cost of trial. The liability of copyright infractions goes beyond an individual. Companies and institutions are more likely to be brought to court than are specific individuals. The company or agency is brought to court for permitting the violation to occur. A perioperative nurse might make an error regarding how materials are used during in-service instruction, in patient education, or on institutional Web sites. Single individuals have been pursued when a professional organization chose to make a public example of the consequences of copyright violation. The safest thing to do is protect yourself with knowledge; know what copyright is, the rights of the specific products with which you are working, and any contracts associated with the use or distribution of these creative works. Keep copies of correspondence and any contracts you have signed.

WAYS TO PROTECT YOURSELF

The first thing to do when using someone else's work is ensure that it is allowed that the material be used in this new way. Contact the copyright holder and ask for permission for this use. If a CC license is identified, check the license for the specific uses permitted.[4] Keep copies of these permissions in case any questions arise. Recall the analogy of the car in attempting to use text, graphics, or programs that have been seen on the Internet. People can look at someone's car but need permission to drive it. **Just because something is viewable on the Internet does not imply that other people can copy the resource.** Ability to look at a graphic on the Internet does not include right to copy and reuse it. Owning a book allows people to have a book, not reproduce the content. Subscribing to a journal or current awareness service allows the subscriber the use of the product as specified by subscription service. Check the contracts for these services. Honest and reasonable attempts to locate the owner/creator of materials should occur if materials are found on the Internet and someone wants to copy and reuse those materials. Do not use materials that do not have explicit permissions for this new use. If reuse is on the Internet, often linking instead of copying is sufficient, because linking is not copying and redistribution.

Linking permits the owner/creator to maintain control of the distribution of the material. If the material is simply linked and not copied and the owner decides not to allow this reuse, the owner can choose to remove the original object. As a linked object, if the owner removes the original, the link is broken and the material is no longer available on the secondary site. Linking to an object maintains the rights of the copyright holder to reproduce, distribute, and display the work as he or she sees fit.

Check the license on computer graphics or other image resources. Just because some graphics are part of a computer program does not mean that reproducing these graphics is permissible. There are some cases where graphics may have been included with purchased software but permission to use these graphics in public forums is not included. Check the contract included with the software or on the product's Web site. If necessary, contact the copyright holder or software company for clarification. Keep copies of these communications. If permissions are not given, consider searching the Internet for similar graphics that are available for use. Creative people (perioperative nurses) can, of course, develop their own.

Photographers hold the copyright for their photographs. The individuals or institutions in the photographs do not have copyright privileges. A health care institution has obligations to protect the privacy of patients and children. An organization may also limit access to items and how the identifiable components are portrayed. Individuals who are photographed may have other options regarding how they are portrayed in these photographs, such as restricting the use to within the hospital for educational purposes only but not beyond that function. Access and portrayals are not related to copyright but rather fall under privacy, trademark, trespass, slander, libel, or other laws. If you are photographing people or physical property for distribution, consider asking permission to do so and keeping copies of these permissions. If you are using someone else's photographs, ensure that you have permission for that use and the use respects the additional laws.

Fair use may permit someone doing a presentation to use graphics and other materials that enhance the presentation. The presentation may fit within the fair use educational use factor. **Change the format of any handouts to include only the text and do not include clip art or other components of the presentation software**. The handouts are for reproduction and distribution. If graphics from nursing textbooks or articles are necessary components, consider obtaining permission to use these graphics.

Sharing articles with a few colleagues or posting a copy on a bulletin board is probably reasonable. Copying an article for a specific patient is also probably reasonable. Reproducing articles or standards of practice for each person in a class, in-service session, group of patients, or research group may be in copyright violation. Consider providing instructions on how these materials may be obtained by the individuals. Buying reprints for distribution is also an option.

SUMMARY

Copyright laws and regulations are complex and have changed over time. There can be significant costs of not recognizing or disregarding these laws. Care in ensuring appropriate use of creative works and keeping documentation can protect the user from some of the risks. There are initiatives to ease the burden of care, increase access to valuable knowledge, and share creative works. CC licenses, open access initiatives, and generous creative people are part of these initiatives.[6,7,8] Consider participating in these initiatives when engaging in creative efforts. When publishing articles, read the author contract and consider author addendums.

REFERENCES

1. US Copyright Office. Copyright law of the United States and related laws contained in Title 17 of the United States Code [circular 92]. Available at: http://www.copyright. gov/title17/. Accessed March 13, 2012.
2. US Constitution, Art 1, Sec 8, Clause 8.

3. US. Copyright Office. Appendix B. The Digital Millennium Copyright Act of 1998. Available at: http://www.copyright.gov/title17/92appb.pdf. Accessed March 13, 2012.

4. Copyright. In S. Phelps, J. Lehman, editors. West's encyclopedia of American law, vol. 3. 2nd edition. Detroit (MI): Gale; 2005. p. 190–200.

5. US National Library of Medicine. Copyright information. Published September 2011. Available at: http://www.nlm.nih.gov/medlineplus/copyright.html. Accessed March 13, 2012.

6. Creative Commons. About. Available at: http://creativecommons.org/about. Accessed March 13, 2012.

7. What is SPARC? Scholarly Publishing and Academic Resources Coalition. Available at: http://www.arl.org/sparc/about/index.shtml. Accessed March 13, 2012.

8. SPARC. Author rights: using the SPARC author addendum to secure your rights as the author of a journal article. Published summer 2006. Available at: http://www.arl.org/sparc/author/addendum.shtml. Accessed March 13, 2012.

9. Harper GK. The TEACH Act Copyright Crash Course. Published 2007. Available at: http://copyright.lib.utexas.edu/teachact.html. Accessed March 13, 2012.

10. Harper GK. Fair use of copyrighted materials Copyright Crash Course. Published 2007. Available at: http://copyright.lib.utexas.edu/copypol2.html. Accessed March 13, 2012.

Spreadsheet and Relational Database Programs:
Useful Tools for Perioperative Nurses

Patricia Newcomb, RN, PhD, CPNP[a,b,]*

KEYWORDS

- Perioperative nurse • Spreadsheet • Relational database
- Evidenced-based practice

KEY POINTS

- Clinicians should be aware that simple spreadsheet programs are usually available on computers in nursing units and can be useful tools for staff nurses.
- In the absence of commercial reference management software, a spreadsheet program can efficiently organize literature for evidence-based projects.
- Simple spreadsheet programs can be used to organize and analyze data collected in research or evidence-based projects.

Information management has become a critical skill for all nurse professionals, including perioperative registered nurses (RNs). In perioperative nursing, combinations of high-touch and high-tech patient needs require staff to be acutely aware clinically. Staff members are focused on responsibilities for assessing, monitoring, and intervening in specific patient situations and may miss the importance of learning to successfully manage amounts of data greater than those generated by one patient at one particular time. When staff nurses and managers begin to think about collecting evidence to demonstrate the quality of their performance or when they begin to express the wish to test their hunches about the factors that influence patient outcomes in their units the time to develop competencies in formal data management has arrived. Fortunately, the challenges of learning to organize and manipulate data do not approach the difficulty of the challenges faced by perioperative nurses in practice on a daily basis.

The author has nothing to disclose.
[a] University of Texas at Arlington College of Nursing, 411 South Nedderman Drive, Lab 119, Arlington, TX 76019, USA
[b] University of Texas at Arlington Genomics Translational Research Lab, Arlington, TX, USA
* University of Texas at Arlington College of Nursing, 411 South Nedderman Drive, Lab 119, Arlington, TX 76019.
E-mail address: pnewcomb@uta.edu

Perioperative Nursing Clinics 7 (2012) 211–221
doi:10.1016/j.cpen.2011.09.001
1556-7931/12/$ – see front matter © 2012 Elsevier Inc. All rights reserved.

Most staff RNs are aware of spreadsheet and database programs loaded onto their workplace computers, but they may not take full advantage of them. These programs can be useful both as practice tools and as repositories of information that may be used in evidence-based projects or research. The current interest in evidence-based interventions to support patient safety and quality care, as well as the movement toward attainment of Magnet recognition in hospitals, mean that perioperative staff RNs serve actively on evidence-based practice and research councils and are participating in clinical research themselves. These activities offer broad scope for common spreadsheet and database programs that are accessible to staff nurses. Staff nurses and managers increase their value to the organization when they learn to use these programs.

PROGRAMS

The term *spreadsheet* refers to lined "sheets," or tables, of rows and columns that have been used in paper form by accountants or bookkeepers for hundreds of years. The columns and rows on a spreadsheet were a way of organizing data so that the user could see how costs, income, taxes, and other items "spread." Traditionally, figures were entered into the columns, and mathematical operations, such as addition and subtraction, were performed manually by the individual entering data into the tables. Row/column financial programs requiring large-scale computer capacity were used in the 1960s, but the first electronic spreadsheet program designed to be used interactively on a personal computer was VisiCalc, developed by Dan Bricklin and Bob Frankston in 1979.[1] Most electronic spreadsheets in use today are direct descendants of VisiCalc.

Currently most health systems use personal computers (PCs) with Windows-based operating systems in patient care units and across most of the system, with the exception of specialized departments such as marketing. Typically, workplace PCs are loaded with Microsoft Office products such as the spreadsheet program, Excel, which seems to be the market leader for electronic spreadsheets presently. In this article the Excel program is assumed to be the default spreadsheet program available to staff nurses.

At first glance, relational database programs look similar to spreadsheets, but they have added sophistication. Commercial relational database programs designed for use on PCs include the Corel Paradox program that is part of the WordPerfect office suite and the Microsoft Access program that is part of Microsoft Office. Like Excel, Microsoft's Access database came to dominate the market for PC-based relational databases. Because most health systems use Microsoft products on computers that are accessible to nurses, it is likely that Access will be available, and that is the database program used as a model here.

A relational database is a system that stores data in tables, like spreadsheets, but a key difference between spreadsheets and relational databases is that the data stored in the relational database can be presented in many different ways, not just rows and columns. Another crucial difference is that, unlike spreadsheets, the data storage tables in a relational database can be linked (related) to each other in different ways. For instance, in a one-to-one relationship, a record in one table is linked to another record in a different table. In a many-to-one relationship, one record in a table is related to many records in another table. Data stored in the tables are organized in a highly structured way that enables queries and the generation of reports. Relational database programs are typically more difficult for practicing

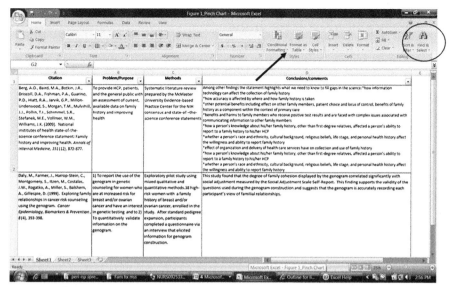

Fig. 1. Pinch chart. Formatting as a table increases functionality and is done easily by selecting the Format as Table option (*arrow*). Note Find feature (*circle*).

nurses to master but offer better means to protect data integrity and better reporting mechanisms than spreadsheets.

SPREADSHEET PROGRAMS IN PRACTICE
Storing Information as Text

Data stored in tables are easily read, retrieved, and manipulated. Spreadsheets make tabulating both text and numerical data easy. As staff RNs become more engaged in evidence-based practice and conduct evidence-based projects supporting such practice, they are consuming greater volumes of research literature. Many staff RNs print out paper copies of articles and store them in file folders, accordion files, or other cardboard-type containers. Recall and retrieval of information from these containers is usually cumbersome.

Commercial reference management software such as RefWorks or EndNotes provides an excellent vehicle for storing citations, generating bibliographies, and preparing manuscripts, but such software may not be available for practicing nurses in the work environment. In the absence of commercial citation management software, spreadsheet programs can be used as "pinch charts" to store and organize critical information from references. A pinch chart is a table containing concise statements regarding critical components of scholarly articles. This type of chart is invaluable as a means of organizing and sharing information from the literature. In a pinch chart, each row in the spreadsheet is a reference such as a journal article, and columns contain the information the user wishes to find rapidly. **Fig. 1** is an example of part of a pinch chart constructed in Excel 2007. An advantage of a spreadsheet pinch chart is that it can be easily customized to suit the nurse's favored ways of tagging or locating information. For instance, information in columns can be sorted, and selected columns can be hidden by the reader when only one kind of information is sought. Columns, rows, and cells can be color-coded, and text can be highlighted.

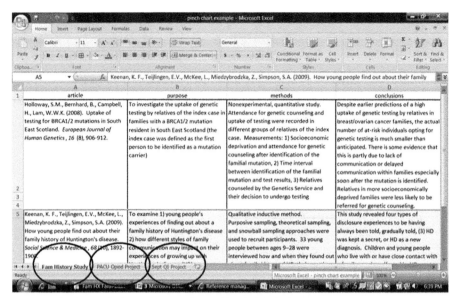

Fig. 2. Multiple pinch charts in a single workbook (*circled*).

Spreadsheet tables have more functionality and are therefore more flexible than tables created in a word processing program.

In Excel, formatting as a table will insert a drop-down menu in each column, which allows quick sorting. This formatting choice will also automatically format cells to wrap text so that each entry can be contained in one cell. This option is especially helpful if the user wishes to cut and paste information into the spreadsheet, although cells can be easily formatted individually as well. Formatting as a table is done easily by selecting the Format as Table option (see arrow in **Fig. 1**) from the Styles section of the menu bar across the top of the spreadsheet. The menu across the top of the page is the Home menu and contains seven sections. The Styles section allows the user to choose conditional formatting, formatting as a table, and cell styles.

If a nurse is seeking a particular author in a lengthy pinch chart, the sorting function can be used to alphabetize the citation column. Additionally, Excel has a Find feature (see circle in **Fig. 1**) on the Home menu, which can be used to find specific words, phrases, dates, and numbers. If specific columns are not of interest they can be hidden by simply selecting the column (at the top) with a right click of the mouse and selecting Hide. Ways of manipulating information in tables and formatting tables are numerous and easy to learn through simple exploration of the menu options. Help is available by clicking the question mark on the menu bar or pressing F1.

Each Excel workbook contains as many worksheets as desired, and this characteristic can be used to advantage for literature storage. For nurses involved in multiple projects, each worksheet may contain literature for separate projects as in **Fig. 2**. In other situations a single workbook might contain separate worksheets for each author or topic contained within a literature review.

Frequently Used Calculations

The formula function in spreadsheet programs is the feature that permits these programs to transcend the simple information storage role. Spreadsheets can be

---

Box 1
Creating a BMI calculator

1. Set up columns on the spreadsheet for each variable including the measurements the nurse will enter and the values that will be calculated. Variables may be in any order, but the figure shows columns ordered in the sequence of the calculation.

2. The first two columns contain height values. Inches or meters will be entered by the nurse.

3. The third and fourth columns contain weight values.

4. To create a formula in a cell, begin by entering the = sign, then type the formula directly into the cell as below.

5. Column E calculates the imperial formula for BMI. The equation is: BMI = [(weight in pounds) · 703] ÷ (height in inches)^2. To command this operation, select cell E2 and type the following: =(C2*703)/(A2*A2). (See **Fig. 3**)

6. Cell names can be entered into the formula by clicking on the target cell.

7. After entering the formula, move the cursor to another cell or press ENTER. The solution to the formula will appear in the formula cell. The formula will remain in the cell until it is changed. Data can be entered repeatedly into the first columns to calculate different BMI values.

8. To limit the number of decimal places in the answer, right-click E at the top of the column and select Format Cells from the drop-down menu. Change category to Number and indicate the number of decimal places you desire.

9. To calculate using metric values in column F, type: =D2/(B2*B2).

---

used to create an enormous variety of calculators that are useful to staff nurses. Although a simple pocket calculator can be used for most calculations of interest to nurses, pocket calculators can perform only one operation at a time, resulting in breaking up some formulas into several steps. Once a formula is created on a spreadsheet, the entire sequence of calculations will be performed instantly when the nurse inserts values of target variables.

For example, body mass index (BMI) is frequently calculated prior to determining drug doses or making decisions regarding risk for obesity. There are two formulas for calculating BMI: the imperial formula, which is based on measurements in pounds and inches, and the metric formula, which is based on measurements in kilograms and meters. In the United States, nurses are often required to calculate BMI from imperial measurements but to record BMI in metric measures. Ideally, this work is performed by the electronic medical record (EMR) itself, but when an EMR is not in use or lacks the function, nurses continue to calculate. This operation requires first calculating the BMI formula, then converting from one system to another. The calculations are straightforward but can be performed instantly on a spreadsheet as described in **Box 1**. **Fig. 3** and **4** illustrate the BMI calculator. Similar calculators can be constructed on the same worksheet for frequently used formulas, such as temperature conversions, body surface area, frequently used drugs, and so forth. Keeping the spreadsheet program running and minimized allows quick access to the calculators.

PROJECT DATA

Evidence-based projects, quality improvement initiatives, and research studies require some system for securely storing and organizing data collected about patients or other subjects. Spreadsheet programs are ideal for this purpose in both practice

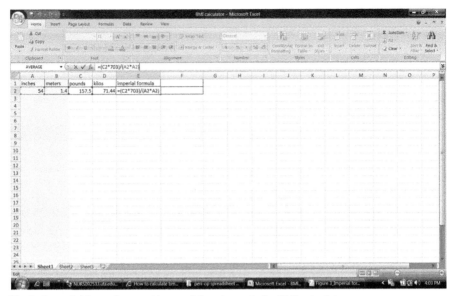

Fig. 3. Imperial formula typed into cell 2, column E, for BMI calculator.

and research situations. Basic statistical analyses can be carried out directly in these programs as noted later, and data stored in Excel can be easily imported into statistical programs for more sophisticated analyses.

For instance, for quality improvement purposes, nurses may desire to collect data regarding patient outcomes. Consider length of stay in the pediatric postanesthesia

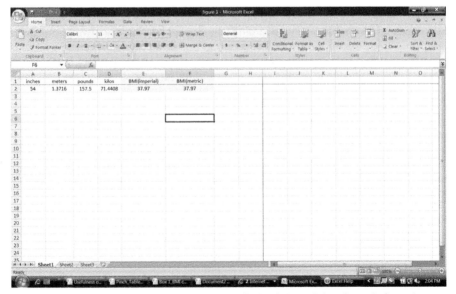

Fig. 4. Completed BMI calculator with solutions for both imperial and metric formulas.

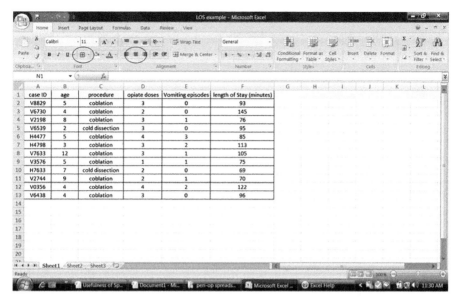

Fig. 5. Example of spreadsheet showing length of stay in postanesthesia following tonsillectomy. Note Gridlines and Center Text functions (*circled*).

unit following tonsillectomy. A nurse wishing to collect these data and data regarding factors that might be related to length of stay can easily do so in a spreadsheet. **Fig. 5** illustrates a spreadsheet with relevant data. Appearance of the table can be easily changed to suit the nurse by using functions such as the Gridlines function (see **Fig. 5,** circled), which highlights the desired lines in the table, or the Center Text function (see **Fig. 5**, circled) for moving cell contents to the center of the cell. When the same value appears in multiple consecutive cells, such as the "coblation" value in the procedure column, the cell contents can be quickly copied by placing the cursor at the right lower corner of the cell to be copied until a black cross appears, then, keeping the left mouse button depressed, dragging the cross down across the cells that are to receive the copied information.

DATA ANALYSIS

Once the nurse has collected the target information in a project, simple arithmetic operations and statistics can be generated using the menu of functions. For instance, in the length of stay example, the nurse wishing to know the average age of subjects can select any cell (but it is reasonable to select the cell under the values in the age column), then click the *fx* (function) icon, which will cause the Insert Function dialog box to appear (**Fig. 6**). In the example, cell B14 has been selected so the formula will be constructed in that cell. The equal sign is generated when the *fx* icon is selected. The nurse can then select Average from the menu list (see **Fig. 6**) and then click OK. This action will cause a Function Arguments dialog box to appear (**Fig. 7**). Because cell B14 was previously selected, the program assumes the average desired is from cells B2 through B13, and the average is displayed in the top field of the dialog box as Number 1. The formula results are displayed in the dialog box. If this is the set of numbers desired to include in the calculation of the average, the nurse has only to click OK. The formula result will now appear in cell B14. In **Fig. 8**, the averages are

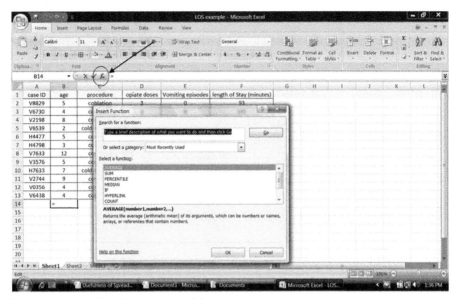

Fig. 6. Inserting a function in a spreadsheet.

displayed for all the pertinent columns and were generated in seconds. If long strings of numbers following the decimal are not desired, select the cell, such as F14 in this example, and select Format Cells from the drop-down menu. Under the Number tab there are multiple choices for the type of display available. The author chose Number and then 2 in the Decimal Places field. A look at the list of functions in the insert

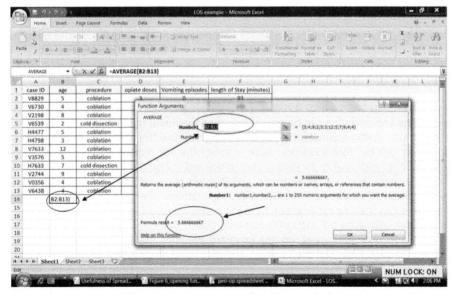

Fig. 7. The arguments dialog box in the process of making a calculation in a spreadsheet.

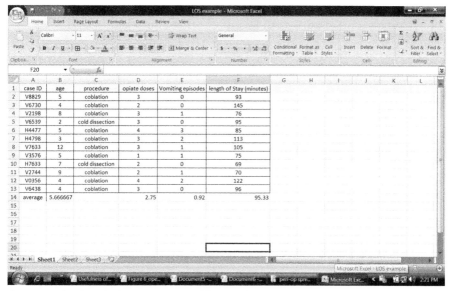

Fig. 8. Result of a calculation in a spreadsheet: column averages.

function dialog box reveals that the spreadsheet program is able to calculate a wide variety of statistics such as standard deviations, t-tests, correlations, and so forth.

RELATIONAL DATABASES IN PRACTICE

The Access database program available in the Microsoft Office suite of programs has been a workhorse for years but has been difficult for occasional users to master. The later versions (post-2007) have simplified the use of the tool, although it is still more challenging than Excel. Other important relational database management systems (RDMs) include Oracle, Apache Derby, CUBRID, Empress Embedded Database, Ingres, and others. Because Microsoft products are those most commonly available on PCs for staff nurses, the Access RDM will be the model in this article.

The first database management systems emerged in the 1970s after Edgar Codd[2] published a report describing the application of elementary relation theory to systems that would provide shared access to large collections of formatted data. To appreciate the relational database, it is only necessary to look at an example of the flat database that preceded it (**Fig. 9**). Flat databases were virtually impossible to search except for reading each data item from the beginning. Contemporary relational databases, which may contain thousands of linked tables of data, are easily searched using a special computer language called Structured Query Language (SQL). When using programs designed for PCs such as Access, the consumer need not

| Lname, Fname, age, diagnosis|ladysmith, Josiah, 12, retinoblastoma |Daniels, Margery, 22, ovarian cyst|Hull, Franklin, 85, hip fracture |

Fig. 9. Flat database. Flat databases preceded relational databases and were virtually impossible to search except by reading each data item from the beginning.

Lname	Fname	Age	diagnosis	physician
Ladysmith	Josiah	12	Retinoblastoma	1
Daniels	Margery	22	Ovarian cyst	4
Hull	Franklin	85	Hip fracture	3

Physician #	Name	Office address	RN/MA contact
1	Gergon	2413 Avenue M	Mary Morgan, RN
2	Howells	3000 River Oaks	Jennifer Ojeda, MA
3	Mancuso	2516 Avenue N	Laurel Gray, RN
4	Wells	4317 Bayless Street	Bill Jones, RN

Fig. 10. Format of tables in an RDMS. The second table is related to the first table through the physician field.

understand SQL. The end user can perform complex tasks without specialized knowledge of computer languages because the sophisticated user interface is generally intuitive and reduces the work to mouse-clicks. The Help icon is also our friend!

Data in an RDMS are stored in tables of columns and rows that look similar to a spreadsheet. The flat database (see **Fig. 9**) would be formatted as in **Fig. 10**, with each row representing a record and each column representing a field. The second table in **Fig. 10** is related to the first table through the physician field. In this example (see **Fig. 10**), all physician information is kept in a table separate from the patient data but can be quickly and easily accessed through the physician number link. For those who are new to Microsoft Access, the newer versions feature "wizards" or introductory videos that walk the user through the creation of tables and the linking process.

Relational databases are extremely useful in situations that require the quick generation of attractive reports. The information in a table (see **Fig. 10**) can be used in multiple different reports. After the tables are linked, reports can be generated in a matter of seconds simply by selecting the fields desired in the report (**Fig. 11**). For the beginner, using the report wizard in Access is easy and definitely the wiser course to avoid frustration. Among other advantages, keeping tables up to date in relational databases makes it possible to present well-organized information in an attractive format for last-minute meetings or impromptu briefings.

More personal uses for desktop relational databases are common. For instance, a nurse manager who keeps information about staff such as T-shirt size, birthdays, hire dates, awards, and so forth in a table in a relational database can quickly generate special-occasion reports for staff celebrations. Because tables are linked, data updates are easy and organization of information is efficient. Information needs to be entered only once in a relevant table to be available for any data manipulation thereafter.

A benefit of relational databases that is not duplicated in spreadsheets is the ability to enforce integrity rules. The rules protect the validity of the data. For instance, if entity integrity is enforced, then every record will have its own specific identify and there will be no duplicated records. Referential integrity means that the user can define "primary" and "foreign" keys, which are fields in tables that act as links between tables. When properly defined, these keys prevent inconsistent deletions or updates. If a record is removed from one table, it will be removed from all tables, and if data are changed or added in one table, the change or addition will be reflected in all relevant tables or reports.

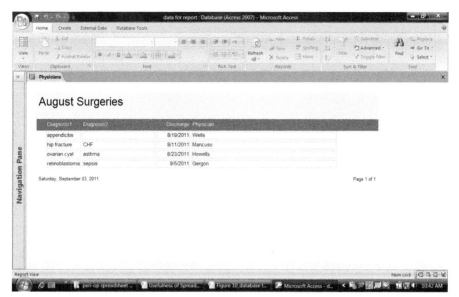

Fig. 11. Report in a relational database. The information in a table can be used in multiple different reports. After the tables are linked, reports can be generated in a matter of seconds simply by selecting the fields desired in the report.

Perioperative RNs who are involved in research or quality improvement projects are probably frequently using spreadsheets. If so, they may have accumulated tens to hundreds of Excel files. At that point, the benefits of a relational database probably outweigh the burden of the extra time spent learning how to use them. Nurse managers are a second group who could realize benefits from learning how to use relational databases. If the training department in an interested nurse's facility does not offer training in spreadsheet and relational database programs, most local community colleges and universities do so through continuing education courses. Furthermore, the abundance of online tutorials is likely to be adequate for getting started with either type of program.

SUMMARY

Although learning the applications described here should not be formidable, there will inevitably be some moments of frustration. Don't give up. These tools will soon be part of general literacy, and their benefits will outweigh the temporary burden of learning. It may help put the project in perspective to remember the challenges faced as student nurses. Are these skills more difficult than mastering manual blood pressure monitoring or hearing heart murmurs for the first time? With a bit of practice, manipulating data can soon be as second-nature as taking blood pressures and auscultating chests. Eventually it will be fun, too.

REFERENCES

1. Bricklin D. VisiCalc: Information from its creators, Dan Bricklin and Bob Frankston. Available at: http://www.danbricklin.com/visicalc.htm. Accessed May 2, 2011.
2. Codd EF. A relational model of data for large shared databanks. Communications of the ACM 1970;13(6):377–87.

Yellow Pages:
It is All About File Management

Joy Don Baker, PhD, RN-BC, CNE, CNOR, NEA-BC

KEYWORDS

- File management • Personal information management • Structure
- Organization

KEY POINTS

- Organizing categories of Personal Information Management system.
- Role of memory relative to file management.
- Purposes for using a Personal Information Management system.
- Example assignment related to collection, storing, and distribution of evaluated Web sites.

File management is one subset of the broader term Personal Information Management (PIM). PIM subsets incorporate Web site bookmarking and e-mail management,[1] "managing appointments, to-do lists, and contact management."[2(p42)] There are five organizing categories of PIM: "hierarchical, flat, linear, spatial, and network."[1(p1)] PIM is the system used to store electronic and tangible (hard copy) materials such as documents, spreadsheets, photos, e-mail messages, books, and magazines[1,3] gathered over time by a perioperative registered nurse (RN).

This article explores organizing categories as a framework for PIM. A brief exploration of the role of memory in PIM and rationale for using a predefined method for storage and retrieval of data are provided. Purposes for using a PIM system identified in this article are related to quality improvement, staff development, and patient and academic education. One application example activity/assignment illustrates the use of file management to gather, store, and distribute evaluated Web sites. Barriers that must be overcome and benefits to PIM are also discussed. Specific implications regarding perioperative nurses and nursing relative to PIM are suggested throughout the article.

The author has nothing to disclose.
College of Nursing, University of Texas at Arlington, Box 19407, 411 South Nedderman Drive, Arlington, TX 76019–0407, USA
E-mail address: jdbaker@uta.edu

Perioperative Nursing Clinics 7 (2012) 223–235
doi:10.1016/j.cpen.2012.02.006
1556-7931/12/$ – see front matter © 2012 Elsevier Inc. All rights reserved.

GROUP INFORMATION MANAGEMENT

Shared materials or social context[1] fall into a separate arena called Group Information Management,[4] and the devices used to access the information are becoming more prevalent as well, such as using an iPhone and pushing the same information into an iPad and desktop computer using a *cloud* system to share data with others. Combining information without being overwhelmed or resulting in a reduction of productivity is a priority key element of future planning by designers and system developers.[1]

PURPOSES OF PIM
Quality Improvement

The system for reviewing an environmental, health, and safety management system is the foundational base connecting all elements of the electronic health record (EHR) activities and processes.[5] A generic management system was identified and necessary to create a series of voluntary environmental standards. Standards such as those used in ISO 14000 provide a model suggesting processes to reduce harmful environmental effects.[6] The use of the Perioperative Nursing Data Set (PNDS) is a perioperative model and provides the language coded for data collection that can be used for quality improvement.

Staff Development

Tracking of personnel attendance at education sessions for in-service or continuing education is one purpose of PIM. It is also important to determine if education is making a difference in the outcomes of the patients, for example, safety initiatives in the perioperative setting such as hypothermia upon admission to the post anesthesia care unit (PACU). The tracking of incidences and related education initiatives may or may not correlate directly, however, without the data one cannot know. Data can provide answers to whether attending an educational session on culture diversity also exploring age-related care makes a difference in outcomes for patients. The RN's receptiveness to information and whether it is new, reinforcement, or so far out of his or her reference field that it holds absolutely no value for him or her must be considered. Cognitive learning must be evaluated as well as the effectiveness of the distribution method. Distribution methods vary from interactive processes to more of the *sage-on-stage* format where there is neither real responsibility nor accountability for self-learning.

Basing the information collection relative to staff development on the PNDS data elements can assist in determining additional learning needs for the perioperative setting staff. For example, identifying the effects of a *just culture* and the changes necessary to cause that to occur while at the same time determining milestones to monitor to maintain the *just culture* are also critical elements for exploration. Generally, if it is not important to the leaders of the system, it will not be a priority for the RN in the system either.

Patient Education

Patient education is similar in nature, as we must be able to articulate the specific outcomes that we wish to achieve and relate those to the PNDS for monitoring the results and feedback from patients. Consider, for example, a patient who is diagnosed with a critical disease in which death will occur without a surgical procedure. The procedure will require significant blood replacement and the patient's religion forbids blood and blood product use. Exploration of data indicating best practices and resources that can be tapped into to assist with this patient are essential. Knowing where these resources are located and who has the rights to access them are two elements for exploration. The ethical principles at work in this scenario are also important to explore as well the frequency of occurrence in the setting. Determining the PIM for patient education and the outcomes related also needs to be connected to the PNDS, as that is a ready tool for coding data for future analysis.

Academic Education

Teaching individuals how to learn and manage their own personal information can be a challenging endeavor. Given that, individuals may have the *filer* or the *piler* type of PIM strategies already at work. One of the outcomes for the Masters N5308 Nursing Informatics course that I teach is to *apply personal skills in use of information technology appropriate to nursing practice, education, and research.* One of the assignments in the course is what we refer to as the *Yellow Pages* assignment (J.D. Baker, Hough H, Yellow Pages assignment for N5308 Nursing Informatics, Unpublished document, University of Texas at Arlington, College of Nursing, Arlington, TX, 2011). In this assignment, Web pages are utilized as the only files, with the exception of the folder summary documents and the Table of Contents document. The process that is taught can apply to other file formats, but to narrow the volume we selected only Web sites. The file management technique is a hierarchical process with forced main topics in which files may be used only once in any part of the compact disc (CD) created by the student (see **Appendices A** and **B**).

Students have indicated that after completing the assignment they plan to clean up their files on their computer or multiple flash drives so they can locate items more readily. They also have indicated the value of this relative to management of their e-mail as well instead of having everything in the Inbox and Sent box. Students have indicated there is value for creating CDs for patient education. CDs are a low-cost means of conveying information to patients. The patients can be assured of the quality of the Web pages or documents housed on the CD because the items have been preevaluated by the RN. Perioperative nurses can use this same process for dissemination of content, relevant sources, instructional materials, and so forth to patients or staff.

ORGANIZING CATEGORIES
Hierarchical System

The hierarchical system is the more common method of PIM, allowing for a logical as well as an intuitive approach. Operating systems such as Windows utilize a hierarchical system to manage and organize files.[1] This hierarchical system uses a series of folders, subfolders, and file names to facilitate the management of the information. This is similar to that of a library subject category system for locating similar references and was a consistent strategy used by participants in a mechanical engineer's study.[7] An example of the hierarchical system in the perioperative setting could be the implementation of a new piece of equipment requiring *education*, *practice sessions*, *servicing* and *cleaning processes*, *budget*, etc. that are the primary or main folder labels. Subsets or subfolders of *education* might be *users* (RNs, Surgeons, Central Service Technicians, Biomedical staff, etc), *training materials*, and *scheduling* (equipment, rooms, sequence, etc). Individual items retained under each of the main or subfolders could be either electronic files or hard copy files such as participant handouts. This hierarchical system, although cognitively oriented, can also be difficult to maintain as the files and project components expand over time.

Flat

The flat system is a method of "assigning tags or attributes to information items."[1(p4)] This is done in social networking systems in which a photograph is posted so *friends* may view it and the individuals within the photograph are highlighted with their associated name(s) identified, thereby *tagging* the image. Attributes assigned to the same photograph could be the event title, location, date, time, etc. Multiple tags may be assigned to a document or file allowing any of the identified tags or keywords to be used to search for an item.[1] Web-based examples of this can be found in these sites "sharing photos (http://www.flickr.com), Web bookmarks (http://del.icio.us), and articles (http://www.citeulike.org)."[1(p4)] An example of the flat system in the perioperative setting might be using the previous scenario of implementing a new piece of equipment; therefore, associated tags might include *handouts, equipment name, vendor*, etc. This process does take time to annotate the items effectively and consistently.

Linear

Linear structures allow for searching based on a particular attribute for comparison with other items in the system. Examples are "the order of words in dictionaries (alphabetical), entries in weblogs (chronological), and incoming email inboxes (chronological)."[1(p6)] The downside to this type of structure is it can lose dimension such as alphabetic dimension of the item while holding another such as chronological order or the reverse.[1] A perioperative example would be maintaining the minutes of the educational sessions for the new equipment listed in chronological order. One has to remember which meeting a particular issue was addressed to be able to locate it in the future. The ability to find the information by product or vendor name could be lost.

Spatial

The computer desktop as a file location is an example of spatial structure. The spatial feature relies on the premise that what is important is on top and allows for quick access.[1] Limitations of this type of PIM system are size of computer monitor, and resulting significant cluttering of the desktop can occur. The spatial memory method can result in poor performance as an information retrieval process.[1] This process can work for perioperative nursing, for example, using the same scenario of the equipment implementation project if on the desktop one main folder is maintained in the spatial method of the computer desktop. A hierarchical system is used for the subset folders. The project is retained on the desktop because of its priority nature, but other methods can be employed to streamline the management of the desktop to avoid clutter. Once the project is completed, the folder on the desktop housing the entire project materials may be either deleted or archived into another storage system location.

Network

The World Wide Web (WWW) is an example of a global network structure. The network type of system allows connections to be made among information elements in an arbitrary fashion.[1] This system has less structure and is easy for the user to get lost.[1] Connections among information elements are made with a Uniform Resource Locator (URL); information then can be connected in a database using the same identifier. One example of this is using bibliographic software such as Endnotes or RefWorks, which can be used to track references such as books and journal articles using a link to a location hosting the actual document.[8] Another example is using the PNDS codes containing formal definitions. If these are converted to a URL as a tag this then allows a search of the various items/data based on that URL within the WWW or database, allowing information to be retrieved for exploration and analysis.

PERSONAL STYLE DEVELOPMENT

Every person and hospital system will have a preferred PIM category style.[1] Variations might range from an individual who prefers a hierarchical system and regularly updates his or her folders, adding, deleting, and editing files. However, others may prefer all information items to reside in a central location such as My Documents on the Desktop.[1] Others may need a chronological process to manage, for example, a sequence within a project.[1] If one is interested in sharing Web bookmarks, then tagging may be the system of choice.[1] No matter the preference choice, there is occasionally a need for restructuring as needs change. To date there is still a need to allow integration of categories of PIM without duplication, creating more layers for data mining purposes that can be specific and relevant to the items searched.

Having access to multiple means of retrieving information particularly may help users as the methods become more integrated in the future. Depending on the system, users must remember document filenames, the date in which it was created, or the tag with which it was associated.[1] In the future, if an individual can remember one PIM system such as file or folder name, date, tag, etc. when searching it may be enough to locate an item. For now, each person selects a PIM method based on individual choice that will work best under the particular circumstances experienced and preferences for record management. For example, if one person is very organized with a clean desk then a hierarchical system might be an option and might be labeled as a *filer.* If the individual is more of a *piler* (a type of short-term memory) then a spatial organization on the desktop may be his or her choice.[9-11] *Spring cleaners* function under the rule of thumb that *out of sight is out of mind.* The *spring cleaner* may either delete old files or add to folders; however, the item(s) are no longer visible, which can reduce the stress of seeing large open files or piles of materials.

ROLE OF MEMORY IN PIM

Three different types of memory play a role in the PIM.[9] The first is *semantic* memory; for example, when retrieving the item or object from the personal databases it is in a textual format such as consistent folder or file name variation theme. The second is *autobiographical* memory and suggests one has had a previous experience with the item. The third is that of *temporal* reference or memory indicating that it was recently accessed, for example, last week.[9] Memory problems develop relative to retrospective issues such as forgetting details, past event, or information acquired in the past.[9] A second memory problem is prospective or failure to remember a future task, commitment, appointment, etc.[9] The final memory issue is action slips that are "short term memory failures, which cause problems for actions currently being carried out, e.g., forgetting why one went upstairs, or losing one's train of thought, etc."[9(p927)]

PIM STRATEGIES/OUTCOMES

Having the intended outcomes or end results in mind can help establish the rationale for one strategy over another. Taking time to think critically regarding how the PIM systems currently in use fit with the vision, mission, and philosophy of both the employer and individual is important. One's personal learning style may influence the selection of system management strategies. Cognitive learning can take place at various points in the process of storing items for future retrieval. The terms used to label a file today may have significant impact on use tomorrow. Color choice can be a part of this process. For example, *Rainbow Folders*[12] is a free download that allows color coding folders to visually assist with storing decisions and retrieval.

FILE TYPES: SKILLS AND ACCESS

There are four types of management related to e-mail, content, Web pages, and interactive sites such as blogs or wikis. As technology continues to explode on the scene, accessing with the appropriate devise requirements varies as much as the diversity within the human population. There are always costs to upgrades and changes and as these adjustments become the standards, a chasm of continuing a class system gap rears its ugly head. When these changes occur, it may also cause the individual to adjust his or her method of PIM.

E-mail Management

E-mail celebrates its 40th birthday in 2011. Ray Tomilison sent the first e-mail message in 1971.[13,14] E-mail has "three key functions in PIM: task management, personal archiving, and contact management."[15(p68)] The primary problem is that e-mail systems do not handle all of the functions well. Leaving the task-related item in the Inbox is one means of handling priority as long as the size of the Inbox is manageable. A large number of messages in the Inbox makes it more difficult to manage and locate specific task-related items.[15] There are three management strategies: (1) folders textually distributing messages based on subject or content; (2) searching; and (3) sorting "for accessing archived information."[15(p71)] The final function of contact management is generally good in e-mail systems; however, it is sometimes difficult to retrieve information as it often takes a manual process to search and identify the relevant contact sought.[15] The use of sender, recipient, and date also provides cues for locating messages in e-mail systems.[15] The user-subjective principles[3] are both similar and different on some levels. The three principles are project *classification, importance*, and *context*.[3] For the project, everything relative to the project would go under this classification. For the importance, filing is based on value to the user. The final one, *context*, indicates that the "information should be retrieved and viewed by the user in the same context in which it was previously used, to bridge the time gap between these two events."[3(p237)] Within the element of *context,* four attributes were identified: *external, internal, temporal*, and *social*.[3] Strasser[14] suggests six key elements for managing e-mail:

1. Handle messages similar to that of traditional inboxes and written communications.
2. Decide what must be done with the message.
3. Manage mailbox size.
4. Back up periodically.
5. Retain messages and attachments as you would other documentation.
6. Monitor for viruses.[(p506)]

If one assumes that between 75% and 80% of the e-mail messages received are classified as spam or junk, then applying the Pareto principle (**Box 1**) or 80/20 rule indicates that 80% of our time when reviewing e-mail is spent with distractors and unproductive time wasters. Missed or forgotten commitments[16] creates another element of the 80% misuse of time. Although scheduling systems such as Microsoft

---

Box 1
Pareto principle

Pareto principle: Vilfredo Pareto's (economist) rule states, "That a small number of causes is responsible for a large percentage of the effect, in a ratio of about 20:80. Expressed in a management context, 20% of a person's effort generates 80% of the person's results. The corollary to this is that 20% of one's results absorb 80% of one's resources or efforts. For the effective use of resources, the manager's challenge is to distinguish the right 20% from the trivial many."

Reprinted from Hafner AW. Pareto's principle: the 80–20 rule, 1–3. Available at: http://www.bsu.edu/libraries/ahafner/awh-th-math-pareto.html.

Outlook do help bring some of the elements together such as e-mail, appointment scheduling, and to a lesser degree task management, they do not help with the vast amount of unnecessary e-mail that one must deal with on a daily basis.

Allen[17] suggests sorting the e-mail content into four categories: Trash, Tickler, Reference, and Action.[17] These categories are not that dissimilar to those identified by Covey,[18,19] which use a chi square (x^2) grid to aid in decision making. Covey's categories are (1) *Urgent* (crises, pressing problem, or deadline driven); (2) *Not Urgent* and important (category in which one should spend the greater portion of the time available); (3) *Interruptive Activities* may have some degree of urgency; however, these are most often someone else's priority; and (4) *Trivial Activities*, which are generally not urgent or important; they represent the time wasters procrastination deluxe opportunity.[18]

Barreau identified five filing systems used by her participants that are related to tasks, topic, time, provenance, and form.[10] She suggests there are "three types of information in the workplace: ephemeral, working, and archived."[10(p307)] "Ephemeral information has a relatively short shelf life, but requires prominent placement in the work space so that it will not be overlooked."[10(p308)] Working information is content used often over a period of time.[10] "Archived information has long-term value but isn't being used in the current work at hand."[10(p308)]

Other File Types

Content-based items are documents (.docx), portable document format (.pdf), spreadsheets (.xlsx), or presentations files (.pptx) that are stored in the PIM system utilized by the perioperative nurse. The same strategies identified earlier may be employed with these items; however, they also may be relevant in more than one location for retrieval purposes. **Format-based** items such as those used with Web page bookmarks or favorites tend to use a flat or tagging system such as that found in http://delicious.com/[1] This also provides a connection by tagging relative to categories and sharing these sites with others. **Interactive-based** are also a Web page format using URLs to identify and locate. Blogs and wikis are examples of such an interactive structure. Blogs provide an opportunity to display information and then allow others to comment on the content, creating dialogue among those accessing the blog. Wikis are designed for collaborative group work where the end product can be edited by all participants having access to the wiki. Managing and tracking iterations of the wiki can present a challenge.

BARRIERS

Information fragmentation[1] can occur particularly as it relates to finding a specific item stored either in diverse unconnected PIM systems or on multiple "devices such as desktops, laptops, cell phones, and personal digital assistants (PDAs)."[1(p11)] Information overload is one component driving the need for efficient and effective PIM systems. Perhaps multitasking such as using the cell phone during a meeting, reading e-mail while driving, etc. is not a good choice. "Multitasking is a terrible coping mechanism"[20] for dealing with information overload and makes people less productive.[20] The second issue with information overload is that it takes a great deal of self-discipline to take control of the information overload.[20] The steps involve the three "F" elements: Focus, Filter, and Forget. These three Fs are similar to Allen's four elements[17] and Covey's quadrants[18] for working with various pieces of information or interruptions. The third issue is that for change to occur the senior level executive sets the behavior and tone for the organization and he or she has the responsibility to set a better example. The productivity level of the entire organization can be affected by information overload and no one can address the issue alone.[20] Multitasking slows us down, taking "up to 30% longer with twice as many errors."[20(p2)]

Storage availability also seems to be an issue, less so today than in the past. Gemmell and colleagues suggest that over a person's lifetime, less the recordings of "videos, a terabyte [of computer space] seems adequate for lifetime, storage."[21(p90)] They suggested "1GB/month for the duration of an 80-year life assuming only modest storage"[21(p90)] needs could be maintained. I do have a few doubts because of the continuing rapid change and the opportunity to manage massive amounts of information. For example, in the late 1980s I thought a 10 MB computer was huge and now we have flash drives that hold 10 to 20 GB that can fit in a small wallet. The key to this concept is to be able to store *everything* no matter the file, format, or original devise location. Search and retrieval become the critical elements. In addition, cost and copyright issues[21(p95)] have a tendency to surface periodically and rights to storage or retrieval become restricted. The underlying issue becomes, "when everything can be captured, easily found, and utilized, it is not clear whether this capability will always be desired and in some cases allowed."[21(p95)] Legal and societal issues[21] "relative to privacy and security implications"[21(p72)] will continue to surface and cause rich dialogue and debate, both in and outside the courts and legislative systems.

BENEFITS

Benefits to the process of collecting everything can be evaluated against the Five Rs identified by Sellen and Whittake[22] as "recollecting, reminiscing, retrieving, reflecting and remembering intentions."[22(p73)] *Recollecting* is the thinking back in detail past experiences or episodic memories.[22] *Reminiscing* is the opportunity to "relive past experiences for emotional or sentimental reasons."[22(p73)] *Retrieving* could be dependent on inferential reasoning such as keywords[22] and identifying alternate properties in which an item might be located, searched, or sorted. "*Reflection* might include examining patterns of past experiences"[22(p73)] similar to what is conducted in a phenomenological study. *Remembering intentions* is the commitment to prospective events; it is future oriented such as "run errands, take medication, and show up for appointments."[22(p74)]

PERIOPERATIVE NURSING IMPLICATIONS

Examples of two folder strategies are offered: one that may fit the practice arena and one that may fit the education arenas (**Box 2**). Consider four primary folders as the starting point for either concept area. For the practice area, those might be labeled Work, Professional Organization(s), Education/Training, and Personal. For the education areas,

---

Box 2
Sample folder outlines for PIM education and practice areas

Education	Practice
Teaching	**Work/Employment**
• N5308 Informatics	• Orthopedic Nursing
• N5382 Health Policy	• Project: Supply Management
	• Project: Patient Safety
Service/Professional	**Professional**
• AORN	• AORN
○ NLC Region V Coordinator	• State Council
○ State Coordinator for TX	• ANA
• ANA	
• TCORN	
Scholarship	**Education/Training**
• Presentations	• Inservices
• Publications	• CEs
• Posters	• Annual Requirements: BCLS, etc
• Grants/Funding	
Personal	**Personal**
• Family	• Family
• Friends	• Friends

Note: Each of the above items represents a folder the bulleted items represent subfolders and may hold multiple subfolder levels within one folder.

while similar, there is a slight variation on theme: Teaching, Service/Professional, Scholarship, and Personal. Under each of these headings or folders, subfolders may be created to help facilitate the PIM for the individual. An example of subfolders for the education area, for example, under the Scholarship folder, might be something like: Presentations, Publications, Posters, and Grants. An example of subfolders relative to the perioperative RN might fall under the Professional Organization(s) such as Association of Perioperative Registered Nurses (AORN) Congress, Committees, Local Chapter, and American Nurses Association (ANA). There could be more subfolders within each of these headings depending on the individual's personal selection, choices, and themes for contextual hierarchy of files.

For managing the files within the folders and subfolders, decisions have to be made regarding how they will be handled, when changes will be made, and the monitoring timeframe. Whether an item be retained for archival purposes or deleted after its purpose has been served becomes the underlying question for decision making with the PIM. Perioperative RNs are generally quality organizers and detailed planners because of the work done in the perioperative setting. This skill can be translated and used in their PIM system development.

SUMMARY

Of the five PIM categorizing systems, hierarchical, flat, linear, spatial, and network, the hierarchical seems to be the most prevalent.[1] The hierarchical system uses folders and subfolders for organization. This could be an alphabetical system or chronological process and has merit for perioperative nurses. This article addressed file management for the purposes of searching and retrieval of data for use and analysis to improve patient care outcomes and patient safety and to address staff issues for quality improvement. Having data that provides the information to support perioperative practice decisions to continue to improve care, finding quality ways to manage and maintain access to the best practice options, and managing the data will contribute to positive outcomes for patients in the perioperative settings.

APPENDIX A: YELLOW PAGES STUDENT ASSIGNMENT*
Goals

The first goal of this assignment is to utilize a systematic and usable tool for evaluating Web sites. Students may use one of the two created by former students: one is qualitative and the other is quantitative in evaluation format. Students may also choose to use one they locate from the Web that resonates more with their own use or create an entirely new one for themselves. The second goal is to use the identified Web site evaluation tool to select sites for inclusion in a personal nursing *Yellow Pages* CD. The student burns the various individual pages onto the CD using appropriate folders for navigating the CD. If the student used a quantifiable evaluation tool, we ask him or her to provide the associated score of each Web site included in the CD. If the student selected a qualitative evaluation tool then we ask him or her to provide information about how each site fared related to the tool. The final goal is to create a CD with detailed files and links related to the predetermined criteria. This assignment assists the student in developing skills in burning a CD for use by other(s) and management of folders and files of data using both internal and external URLs.

Content Elements

Content areas that must be addressed by the student include creating (1) a Table of Contents linking to the internal pages within the CD; (2) a copy of the Web site evaluation tool employed in the CD; (3) an introduction that is an overview of the organization of the CD and rationale for key themes developed in the folders (sections); and (4) four main folders: Nursing Practice, Education, Research, and Personal Growth/Other. Within the Nursing Practice folder, students are required to demonstrate their skill in creating subfolders. Each folder and subfolder created follows the same principles of quality outline formatting; in other words, there must be a minimum of two under each heading (folder) identified. Therefore, if a student selects to use two subfolders, for example, under Nursing Practice, then there must also be a minimum of two Web page files within each subfolder. The student must also include a summary of what is included in each folder/section explaining how he or she used the evaluation tool to select the specific Web sites included and how the Web sites selected will help you in your practice or relate to the personal value and use.

There are a few *DO NOTs* in the guidelines for this assignment.

1. Do not include materials you consider to have little value and no direct relationship to your practice.

---

*From Baker JD, Hough H. Yellow Pages assignment for N5308 Nursing Informatics. Unpublished document, University of Texas at Arlington, College of Nursing. Arlington, TX.)

2. Do not duplicate Web sites for multiple folders. If a site fits more than one folder/section, please select the best fit and that is where it needs to go.
3. Do not include just a list of URL addresses; you may indicate there are ones you wish to visit in the future but all data should have been evaluated by you.

Testing and Dissemination of the CD

On an individual *Yellow Page,* the student must ensure that each URL address link is active in the CD and will open the associated external Web site. On the Table of Contents students will use internal links within the CD to redirect to the folders, subfolders, and individual *Yellow Pages.* They will use the print screen function to capture a screen shot of each Web page to record with their annotation, tool use, and the URL (see **Appendix B**). In addition to the creation of the *Yellow Pages* CD, students in this course also create and post to the class discussion board their *Top Five* Web sites and annotation of each. This provides the class a comprehensive bibliography of Web sites evaluated by their peers on a variety of subjects. The final part of this assignment is the presentation of the *Top Three* Web sites and showcasing their *Yellow Pages* CD, which allow the students to practice their presentation skill.

Outcomes

With this one assignment, students create a PIM for Web sites they find relevant, learn how to burn a CD for use by someone else, generate an executive summary document we call the *Top Five*, and deliver a presentation to enhance their skills. Their choices of sites to include will depend on the purpose and themes they have selected for the CD. Other associated benefits are that the students begin to see the relevance of managing other information in a conscious, critically thought out method.

APPENDIX B: EXAMPLE YELLOW PAGE WEB SITE

Italics below are notes/instructions about the process and are *not* included in the *Yellow Page* document. Please do not use this Web site in your *Yellow Pages.*

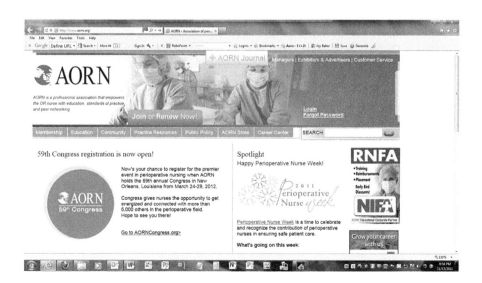

AORN: http://www.aorn.org/

Score/Analysis using Web Evaluation tool: *Insert the score such as 96/100; 1of 5 with 1 high; or evaluation outcome from the tool you selected on each websites document. The evaluation outcome will depend on which tool was selected.*

Create an Annotated note about the site:

AORN is an organization of Perioperative Registered Nurses. The site provides Educational offerings scheduling and the tab I most often frequent is Public Policy as that provides contact information and indicates the pertinent content relative to health care policy initiatives by AORN and being followed by AORN. There is a nice internal search engine that allows searching of the site for example by typing in Congress the materials for the annual convention opens. I placed the home page as the hyperlink and the print screen below instead of showing only the Public Policy webpages to provide the overview of what the site can offer.

REFERENCES

1. Vassileva I, Vassileva J. a review of organizational structures of personal information management. J Digit Inf 2008;9(1):1–19.
2. Teevan J, Jones W. Personal Information Management. Commun ACM 2006;49(1): 40–3.
3. Bergman O, Beyth-Marom R, Nachmias R. The user-subjective approach to personal information management systems design: evidence and implementations. J Am Soc Inf Sci Technol 2008;59(2):235–46.
4. Erickson T. From PIM to GIM: personal Information Management in group contexts. Commun ACM 2006;49(1):74–5.
5. Strasser PB. Management file. Environmental, health, and safety management systems and auditing programs—part II. AAOHN J 2003;51(8):327–30.
6. Strasser PB. Management file. Environmental, health, and safety management systems and auditing programs: part I—the evolution. AAOHN J 2003;51(4):161–3.
7. Hicks BJ, Dong A, Palmer R, et al. Organizing and managing personal electronic files: a mechanical engineer's perspective. ACM Trans Inf Syst 2008;26(4):23:21–3:40.
8. Ovadia S. Internet connection: managing citations with cost-free tools. Behav Soc Sci Libr 2011;30:107–11.
9. Elsweiler D, Ruthven I, Jones C. Towards memory supporting personal information management tools. J Am Soc Inf Sci Technol 2007;58(7):924–6.
10. Barreau D. The persistence of behavior and form in the organization of personal information. J Am Soc Inf Sci Technol 2008;59(2):307–17.
11. Boardman R, Sasse MA. Stuff goes into the computer but doesn't come out: a cross-tool study of personal information management. Paper presented at the Proceedings of CHI, April 24–29, 2004.
12. Rainbow-Folders. Available at: http://www.freewarefiles.com/Rainbow-Folders_program_5495.html. Accessed February 21, 2012.
13. Butler KM. Email celebrates 40th birthday: is it getting better with age? Employee Benefit News 2011;25(10):17.
14. Strasser PB. Management file. Electronic mail communication—management strategies. AAOHN J 2003;51(12):504–6.
15. Whittaker S, Bellotti V, Gwizdka J. Email in Personal Information Management. Commun ACM 2006;49(1):68–73.
16. Denning PJ. The profession of IT managing time [opinion]. Commun ACM 2011;54(3): 32–4.
17. Allen D. Getting things done: the art of stress-free productivity. New York: Penguin; 2001.

18. Covey SR. The seven habits of highly effective people: restoring the character ethic. New York: Simon & Schuster; 1989.
19. Covey S, Merrill A, Merrill R. First things first: to live, to love, to learn, to leave a legacy. New York: Simon & Schuster; 1994.
20. Dean D, Webb C. Recovering from information overload. McKinsey Q 2011;(1):80–8.
21. Gemmell J, Bell G, Lueder R. My Life Bits: a personal database for everything. Commun ACM 2006;49(1):88–95.
22. Sellen A, Whittaker S. Beyond total capture: a constructive critique of Lifelogging. Commun ACM 2010;53(5):70–7.

A Virtual Learning Environment for Perioperative Continuing Nursing Education

Toni McKenna, DNSc, RN[a],*, Sarah Jones, MA, MLS[b]

KEYWORDS

- Second Life • Continuing nursing education • Virtual world • Distance education
- Virtual learning environment

KEY POINTS

- Second Life is a virtual-world learning environment that can serve as a venue for creative and engaging continuing nursing education.
- A virtual world is an on-line, three-dimensional graphical, multimedia environment where individuals are represented by avatars (digital versions of self).
- Clinical educators in all nursing and healthcare specialties should be aware of the advantages and many potential uses of Second Life.

Exploring new worlds and creative approaches to delivering continuing education is an adventure worth taking! The basic requirement of content that advances the skills and abilities of the registered nurse (RN) can be met in a number of ways. What is clear though is that continuing education is most effective when the experience fully engages learners, expands their skills and knowledge, provides expert information and opportunity for networking, and entices them to learn more.[1] This article describes how a virtual-world learning environment (Second Life, or SL) was used as a venue for an interactive and creative continuing nursing education activity and the positive outcomes that were achieved for the participants (**Fig. 1**).

CHALLENGES OF CONTINUING EDUCATION

Planning and providing continuing nursing education for specialty nursing groups can be challenging. There are time and space constraints as well as difficulties relieving

The authors have nothing to disclose.
[a] Center for Continuing Nursing Education, University of Texas Arlington, PO Box 19197, 140 West Mitchell Street, Arlington TX 76019, USA
[b] Digital Library Services, University of Texas at Arlington Library, PO Box 19497, 702 Planetarium Place, Arlington, TX 76019, USA
* Corresponding author.
E-mail address: tmckenna@uta.edu

Perioperative Nursing Clinics 7 (2012) 237–250
doi:10.1016/j.cpen.2011.10.001
1556-7931/12/$ – see front matter © 2012 Elsevier Inc. All rights reserved.

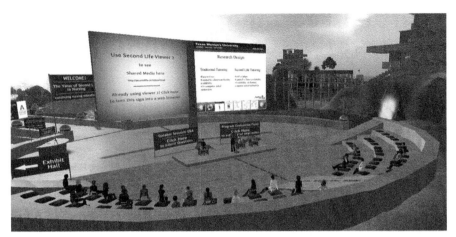

Fig. 1 The University of Texas at Arlington continuing nursing education conference workshop. (*Courtesy of* Sarah Jones.)

staff from their clinical responsibilities, providing adequate depth and applicability of the content, building and maintaining clear learning objectives, and securing expert presenters at the time and place needed. One major obstacle is fully engaging the nurse participants; the education must be impactful, making a difference in their knowledge and practice, and it needs to keep their interest. All of these aspects must occur in a relatively short time frame and at a very reasonable cost, given work and home time constraints and average attention span![2] Finding new and different ways to deliver continuing nursing education can have positive impacts on the quality of the education, the willingness and interest of the professional nurse, and the potential positive outcomes on patient care. The expense of travel and additional time to bring experts together to share their knowledge are further obstacles to providing continuing education. Use of a virtual world as the venue for continuing education can be one of the mechanisms for meeting these challenges.[3]

WHAT IS A VIRTUAL WORLD?

Virtual worlds connect people online in an immersive, engaging way that webcams, Skype, and Web conferencing alone cannot achieve. A virtual world is an online, three-dimensional (3-D) graphical, multimedia environment where individuals are represented by avatars (digital versions of the self). Characteristics of a virtual world[4] include both synchronous and persistence elements.

Synchronousness

Synchronousness means that all participants at a location experience the same environment including the visual scene; the other participants in the form of their avatars; public text and voice chat; the animations of objects or avatars; sounds that come from the environment, objects in the environment or other avatars; and any public multimedia, including Web displays, that are in the environment. Additionally, any changes to the environment happen in real time, and those changes are observable in real time by all participants at the location. Synchronousness allows for live, dynamic demonstrations; participation in and observation of simulations and role-play; and real-time, dynamic, participatory activities in general.

Persistence

Persistence means the environment persists even though a participant has left the location; that environment continues to exist without the necessity of the participant or other avatars being present in the virtual space. Persistence does not necessarily equate to staticness. Persons with the appropriate rights to alter the environment can introduce changes to the environment, which are then observable when a participant returns to that location.

WHY IS A VIRTUAL WORLD A GOOD CHOICE FOR PERIOPERATIVE CONTINUING NURSING EDUCATION?

Using a virtual world to deliver education content offers the opportunity for benefits beyond what Web conferencing or other online platforms can provide. Many online platforms can address issues related to travel and attendant time and cost to participants plus overhead expenses for use of a physical facility. In addition, online platforms allow a participant access to a global range of speakers, discussion groups, and professional networking opportunities. A virtual world, however, adds facets to the experience that other online platforms cannot: sense of self, sense of place, and sense of presence, which derive from the nature of the platform itself. Therefore, a 3-D real-time shared experience can support and reinforce visually, aurally, and interactively the specific purpose and goals of the activities to be carried out. This 3-D immersive environment is combined with "being there" as an avatar with all other participants who are also present in avatar form. Together this experience leads to engagement that other online platforms cannot attain.[5]

Sense of Self

When a person is logged into a virtual world, that person is represented by an avatar that is highly customizable. Virtually all aspects of an avatar's appearance can be changed, from the size and shape of dozens of individual body parts to skin tone and shading, hair style and color as well as a vast range of choices available for avatar clothing and accessories (**Fig. 2**). As a result, it is possible to create a finely tuned representation of the self that reflects what the actual person wishes to project.[6] Crafting this avatar to a person's preferences and experiencing the virtual world through that avatar leads to the sense that the avatar is the person directing it—avatar as self rather than a separate "other."

Sense of Place

The 3-D, multisensory, realistic environment of a virtual world where a person is present as an avatar is key to providing an immersive experience. While embodied in the avatar, the person moves through virtual space and experiences virtual versions of objects, buildings, and outdoor scenes in a way that resembles, and then becomes analogous to, physical-world spaces. With the addition of community (others whose avatars also are present in the space), virtual world spaces become "third places" (gathering places, defined or casual, where people go to be in a social environment).[7]

Sense of Presence

Being an avatar in a 3-D immersive environment together with others who are similarly represented as avatars and sharing real-time interpersonal communication and the same visual and aural experiences in that environment leads to a sense of actually being there.[8] An extension of this sense is the concept of "copresence," which describes avatar embodiment in a 3-D immersive, realistic, space in combination with

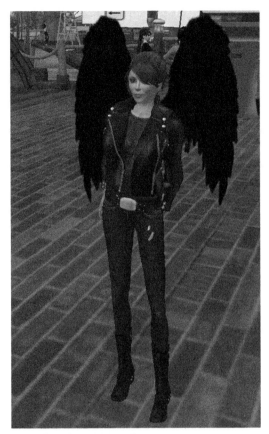

Fig. 2 Avatar in SL. (*Courtesy of* Sarah Jones.)

virtual face-to-face communication with others similarly embodied and is the sense that one is actually present with others despite the physical distance between them (**Fig. 3**).[9]

WHAT IS SL?

SL[10] is a virtual-world platform created and owned by Linden Lab.[11] SL opened to the public in June 2003. Over the 8 years of its existence, SL has been adopted as a platform for learning and outreach by hundreds of universities, colleges, schools, and libraries throughout the world.[12]

User statistics from Linden Lab for the first quarter of 2011 report 794,000 average monthly repeat logins, a rate that was stable over the October 2009 through March 2011 (fourth quarter 2009–first quarter 2011) reporting period.[13] Typically, approximately 58,000 users are logged in at any given time. Whereas other virtual worlds have been used for nonrecreational purposes including World of Warcraft[14,15] and Active Worlds,[16] what distinguishes SL is that user-created content is at its foundation. As a result, it is possible to craft an environment on the SL platform to meet the specific needs of a given purpose. The combination of (1) online platform, (2) overcoming the barriers of distance and travel, (3) synchronous experience for

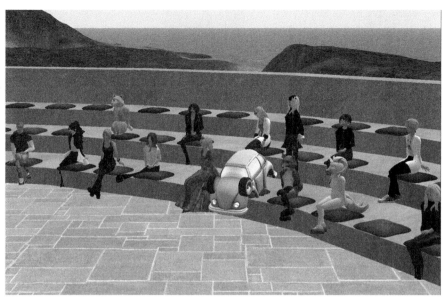

Fig. 3 Participants in SL session. (*Courtesy of* Sarah Jones.)

participants, (4) embodiment and sense of presence from using an avatar in a 3-D shared space, and (5) highly customizable environment has encouraged adoption of the platform by education programs in the United States and internationally.

A sampling of existing uses of SL for nursing and health care:

- *University of Texas (UT) at Arlington College of Nursing Genomics Journal Club.* Since September 2010, the Genomics Journal Club, led by the UT at Arlington College of Nursing Genomics Translational Research Lab[17] science director, Dr Patricia Newcomb, has met in SL as well as face-to-face.[18]
- *US Department of Veterans Affairs military amputee support.* The Telemedicine and Advanced Technology Research Center (Fort Detrick, MD, USA), in partnership with ADL Company (Bloomington, MN, USA) and Virtual Ability, Inc (Aurora, CO, USA), have used an SL-like virtual environment to address peer support needs of military amputees.[19]
- *T2 Virtual PTSD Experience.* The National Center for Telehealth and Technology (T2), a component center of the Defense Centers of Excellence for Psychological Health and Traumatic Brain Injury and part of the Military Health System, has created an environment that incorporates simulations and information to educate visitors about combat-related posttraumatic stress disorder (PTSD).[20]
- *Virtual Hallucinations.* This simulation of a hospital unit incorporates audio and visual elements based on the hallucinations of patients with schizophrenia. Developed as a pilot project, Yellowlees and Cook [21] found that the simulation helped visitors feel that they gained better understanding of auditory and visual hallucinations after touring the environment.
- *The Vanderbilt University School of Nursing.* Through a pilot program, the Vanderbilt University School of Nursing is using an SL environment to prepare faculty to manage clinical simulations with their students.[22]

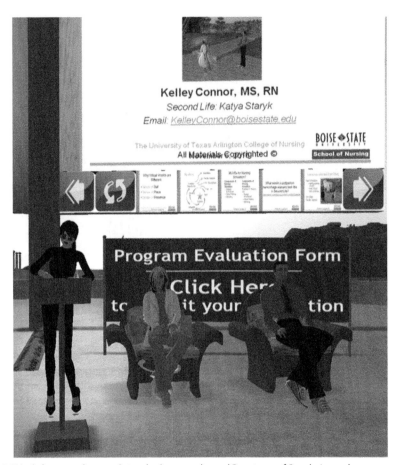

Fig. 4 Workshop moderator introducing speakers. (*Courtesy of* Sarah Jones.)

DELIVERING A NURSING CONTINUING EDUCATION WORKSHOP IN SECOND LIFE

In fall 2010, a nursing continuing education workshop (**Fig. 4**) was held in the virtual world SL through the UT at Arlington Center for Continuing Nursing Education. This workshop was a proof-of-concept project to demonstrate that SL is a platform that can support a quality continuing education experience for nurses to gain multiple benefits without the additional travel time and expense.

The workshop was organized by a planning team, led by Dr Joy Don Baker, which consisted of students in the graduate-level nursing informatics course at the UT Arlington College of Nursing, the Director of the UT Arlington Center for Continuing Nursing Education, the UT Arlington nursing librarian, and the UT Arlington SL coordinator. The planning team was responsible for establishing the learning goals of the workshop, recruiting speakers, setting up the venue, organizing tasks and support roles for the workshop itself, organizing a prework-shop orientation for attendees, promoting the workshop, and ensuring that continuing education units were properly distributed.

The topic chosen for this workshop was The Value of Second Life to Nursing. The team anticipated that most attendees would not be familiar with SL, the current education and health care programs offered there, or the particular characteristics of SL that make it a good place for education and health care activities, thus this choice of topic. The program for the workshop consisted of two presentations: viewing of poster session displays of nursing research and an optional tour of a simulation lab in SL. The simulation lab activity was led by one of the workshop speakers. Learning objectives for the workshop were as follows:

At the completion of this educational activity, the participant will be able to:

1. Define virtual learning environments as they relate to nursing education.
2. Recognize the benefits and challenges of using virtual learning environments for continuing nursing education.
3. Identify the key elements for providing continuing nursing education in any environment.

A Web site[23] was created to accomplish three things: (1) to provide information for prospective and registered attendees, (2) to provide a means for collecting online registrations, and (3) to support publicity efforts for the workshop. Collecting online registrations was important for two reasons. One was simply to know approximately how many people would be attending so that the team could be sure to accommodate the number. Second, preregistration was required for an RN attendee to be able to collect continuing education units upon completion of the workshop. Finally, the registration process included having attendees indicate whether they would be attending a preworkshop orientation to SL. This information allowed the team to plan with Virtual Ability Island staff to provide an optimal orientation experience.

As an adjunct to the workshop, the team provided an opportunity for researchers to set up poster session–type displays of their nursing-related studies. In turn, workshop attendees optionally viewed these displays on a self-guided tour. The

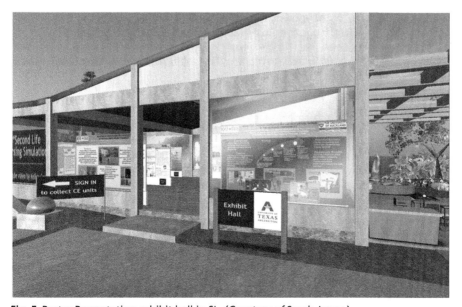

Fig. 5 Poster Presentation exhibit hall in SL. (*Courtesy of* Sarah Jones.)

exhibiting researchers were not required to be present to discuss their research. The team set up an exhibit hall (**Fig. 5**) adjacent to the conference center auditorium for the purpose of housing these displays.

CONSIDERATIONS FOR HOSTING AN EVENT IN SECOND LIFE

As with hosting an event in a physical-world location or using another online platform such as Web conferencing software, there are logistic considerations that will lead to success with hosting an event in SL. These considerations have to do with (1) features of the event venue, including the location of the event, the features of the virtual land, and the design and usability of the venue buildings; (2) services to support both speakers and event attendees, including preevent orientation and training in the SL software and speaker presentation equipment; and (3) planning designed to make the event itself run smoothly including publicity, preregistration for attendees, support staff for the event, and a process for awarding contact hours to RN attendees. Planning and early ongoing evaluation of each of these elements was an important part of preparation. The logistic elements are described in the following sections.

The SL Location

The SL platform uses the metaphor of land to define the virtual environments created within it. Associated with this virtual land are technological affordances and limitations that correspond to the computing resources available on the host servers of the platform. Awareness of the limits, in particular, will allow for creating an environment that will support a successful event.

The Land

In order to maximize the server resources available and to minimize distractions introduced by virtual neighbors, it is recommended that the event be located on a segment of virtual land called a private region, the primary segment of virtual land offered on the SL platform. With one private region an event can comfortably accommodate 30 to 50 attendees, although the limit for the number of avatars per region is 100. For a larger group or to provide a maximally comfortable experience for speakers and attendees, two contiguous private regions can be used, with the workshop location spanning the two regions. This feature allows the event itself to use the server resources of two regions.

The Venue

Although an environment in SL can be created to look like anything from a wheat field[24] to a city[25] or even a fully functional surgical suite,[26] it can be helpful for attendees if the space for a continuing education workshop resembles a location they would expect to visit in the physical world. For this workshop, the team designed a conference center consisting of an open-air auditorium and an adjacent building to house poster session exhibits. Features of the conference center included the following:

- Seating for 60 attendees, with animations to help them control their avatar movements
- Adequate space to allow avatars to move freely
- An architectural design without obstructed views
- Directional signage
- Other signage to help participants understand the function of various objects and locations, including the continuing education sign-in desk.

The adjacent exhibit hall accommodated 11 poster session displays, including a multimedia presentation authored by one of the workshop speakers. Because this multimedia presentation included sound, the team used one of the SL features to prevent that display from disturbing the workshop participants by isolating the display's sound while still having it placed in the exhibit hall along with the other poster session displays. The team chose to use two private regions and to have the main auditorium span the two regions. This configuration allowed the team to have available the server resources of both regions for the event.

Optimizing Technology Performance

In designing a venue, there are steps that can be taken to minimize the server resources required for the event. This optimization helps attendees who may have slower Internet connections or less powerful computers. The steps included minimizing the number of scripts that were used to introduce interactivity into the environment and using best practices such as in the construction of the venue. It is also possible for the manager of the virtual land to remotely restart the server on which the private region resides. Restarting the server additionally helps to ensure a smooth technology experience for the event.

Attendee Orientation

Although some attendees may be experienced in using SL, others may be new to the platform. Therefore, initial training and orientation can optimize the experience. Analogous to these virtual provisions are new members' or first-time attendees'

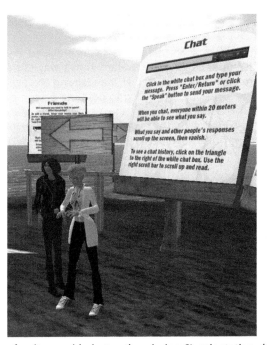

Fig. 6 UT Arlington faculty provide instruction during SL orientation. (*Courtesy of* Sarah Jones.)

tracks, events, and orientations (**Fig. 6**) offered at conferences in the physical world. Helping individuals new to virtual worlds designed for learning allows for more of their time to be spent actually engaged in the learning experience rather than just in venue management.

The team used a preexisting orientation program that is part of Virtual Ability Island,[27] which provides a succession of self-directed tutorial stations. The tutorial stations each address a specific skill needed to navigate the virtual world, for example walking and flying, chatting, animating the person's avatar, customizing avatar appearance, and getting and using new items including clothing and other avatar accessories.

The team's workshop participants were met by a group of Virtual Ability mentors who led attendees through the tutorial stations and provided both small group and one-on-one assistance. An hour and a half was allotted to the preworkshop orientation session. Offering a preworkshop orientation session accomplishes three things:

- It encourages attendees to log in to SL at least once before the workshop.
- It provides a structured opportunity for attendees to become familiar with the SL software.
- Attendees are better prepared to take full advantage of the educational offerings that the workshops provide.

Support for Speakers

As in a physical venue, speakers in a virtual world need to have logistic and technology support for their presentations. The SL analog for this support differs in the specific implementations of this support in two areas (1) ease of use and (2) multimedia presentation tools.

Ease of use

At the conference center location in SL, the team provided dais seating for the presenters and moderators. Seating the avatars in this way put each avatar into a predetermined, appropriate animation rather than leaving the avatar open to extraneous movements that would be distracting to both the person directing the avatar and the participants who were watching the scene on their computer screens. Similarly, the team provided a podium with an appropriate animation so that the speakers could focus on their talk rather than be distracted by unintended movements of their avatars.

Multimedia presentation tools

The team provided two types of presentation tools. The primary tool was a screen for PowerPoint-type presentations in SL. With this tool, a presentation could be created using standard presentation software, with the individual slides saved as a separate image. The presentation screen tool allowed for group viewing of the slides as well as letting the presenter move forward and backward through the slide set. The second tool was a media-enabled object designed to function as a Web browser. Web pages displayed on this object were viewable in real time by all participants at the location. In addition, the presentations were browsable by participants at the location. Links on a Web page displayed on this object were clickable by participants at the location, Web pages were scrollable, and all participants at the location could observe this Web browsing in real time. This media-enabled object allowed the speakers to display Web-based multimedia as part of their workshop presentations.

Event Support Staff

The team also arranged for the event to have a variety of support staff to ensure a smoothly running workshop. The support staff included five specific roles: moderator, greeters, sign-in registrar, transcribers, and event manager.

Moderator

A person from the planning team was designated the moderator for the event. This person introduced the speakers, kept track of timing, facilitated the transition between speakers, and moderated the question-and-answer session that followed the main presentations.

Greeters

Two other individuals functioned as greeters to help attendees know where to go and what to do as they arrived at the workshop.

Sign-in registrar

To meet the requirements for distributing contact hours awarded to preregistered RNs for attending the workshop, one individual was assigned the task of taking and verifying registration. This function allowed the planning group to verify attendance of the participants.

Transcribers

SL supports two methods of public communication: text chat and voice chat. The SL software will print text chat into a nearby chat window for a person to read and review. However, for presentations like the ones in this workshop, using voice chat is easier for the presenter (avoiding the effort, typographic errors, and time delay of typing passages of text) and easier for the attendee, with attendees listening in a way that is comparable to a physical world venue. However, to accommodate those who for technological or other reasons are not able to listen to the presentation, the team provided voice-to-text transcribers. One transcriber was assigned to each of the two presenters, and a third transcriber was assigned to the moderator. Besides accommodating those unable to listen to the voice presentations, having transcribers allowed for individuals to have a text record of what was said at the workshop. The SL software allows for saving text chat to a file on the participant's computer.

Event manager

An event manager was on hand to provide support for various SL technical functions and also generally to watch out for potential difficulties during the workshop.

Publicity

The planning group took advantage of a variety of publicity opportunities to encourage participation by both current SL residents and nurses new to SL. Among these opportunities were e-mail lists specifically for education uses of SL: the SL Educators mailing list[28] and the Healthcare Support and Education mailing list.[29] Notices publicizing the event were sent to those e-mail lists in addition to other, physical-world–based methods of promotion.

Awarding Contact Hours

As with any continuing nursing education activity, early planning is the key to success. During the planning, the objectives were identified, content was outlined clearly, and exact number of minutes of the actual educational activity were calculated. In compliance with the 60-minute per contact hour standard, this virtual world activity provided 1.0 contact hour for the nurse participants. Once attendance was verified, each participant received a completion certificate by e-mail.

OUTCOMES OF THE WORKSHOP

Thirty-one individuals attended the workshop. Of these, 19 RNs received the 1.0 contact hour certificate for their attendance, and the 5 non-RNs received certificates of attendance. Ten others attended who did not preregister and did not receive contact hours or certificates of attendance. Eleven RNs and 2 non-RNs preregistered but did not attend the workshop. Of the 19 RNs who received contact hours, 1 was located in New Zealand, 1 in Massachusetts, and 1 in North Carolina, and the rest were located in Texas. The attendees in Texas included 3 in locations distant from Arlington: 1 in Brownsville, 1 in Allen, and 1 in Spring. Of the 5 non-RNs who received certificates of attendance, 1 was located in Poland, whereas the rest were in the Arlington area.

Although the number of participants was not large, the responses of the 19 RNs and their evaluative feedback were very important. Evaluation was done electronically using a common survey tool. All participants were told in advance that they needed to verify their attendance and complete the evaluation form in order to receive their completion certificate with contact hours.

Overall, participants reported that they achieved the learning objectives and were highly satisfied with the educational experience. Most important, when asked how they would integrate what they learned from this activity into their practice, they responded with specific comments including, "Will look to implement SL activities into my advanced physical assessment course, introduce SL as an alternate continuing education option for staff, explore use in nursing education."

Participants found that the most valuable parts of the activity included visiting the second-floor critical care unit during the activity, having the speakers share their experiences with virtual world leaning, and ability to practice in the New Zealand SIM lab. One participant found that the running chat during the session where the transcribers were capturing the speakers talk was distracting. Other than that, there were no negative comments about the activity, the speakers, the content, or the venue. Participants seemed to benefit from the orientation session that was offered and had very little difficulty learning how to actively participate in the educational session based on the feedback they provided in the evaluation data.

SUMMARY

Providing continuing nursing education in a way that fully engages the learner and offers valuable skills and knowledge that nurses can apply to their work will always be a challenge. Realizing that there is a need for both sufficient time and planning prior to an event is essential. Using a virtual world as the venue for such continuing education offers many advantages such as no need for travel, a sense of being present, and real-time communication with participants. This learning environment can be an exciting and meaningful adventure to undertake for both participants and educators!

REFERENCES

1. Dealey MF, Bass M. Professional development: factors that motivate staff. Nurs Manage 1995:26(8):32F-32I.

2. Schweitzer DJ, Krassa TJ. Deterrents to nurses' participation in continuing professional development: an integrative literature review. J Contin Educ Nurs 2010:41(10): 441–7.
3. American Nurses Association, National Nursing Staff Development Organization. Nursing professional development: scope and standards of practice. Silver Springs (MD): American Nurses Association and National Nursing Staff Development Organization; 2010.
4. Bell MW. Toward a definition of "virtual worlds." Journal of Virtual Worlds Research 2008;1:(1). Available at: http://journals.tdl.org/jvwr/article/view/283/237. Accessed September 11, 2011.
5. Mayrath MC, Traphagan T, Jarmon L, et al. Teaching with virtual worlds: factors to consider for instructional use of Second Life. Journal of Educational Computing Research 2010;43:(4):403–44.
6. Sung Y, Moon JH, Kang M, et al. Actual self vs. avatar self: the effect of online social situation on self-expression. Journal of Virtual Worlds Research 2011;4:(1). Available at: http://journals.tdl.org/jvwr/article/view/1927/3044. Accessed September 15, 2011.
7. Peachey A. The third place in Second Life: real life community in a virtual world. In: Peachey A, Gillen J, Livingstone D, et al. editors. Researching learning in virtual worlds (human-computer interaction series). London: Springer; 2010. p. 91–110.
8. Whang EW, Taylor K, Cash T. Education and virtual worlds: how identity and presence affect users' experience. In: Tettegah S, Calongne C, editors. Identity, learning and support in virtual environments (educational futures: rethinking theory and practice), vol. 36. Rotterdam (The Netherlands): Sense Publishers; 2009. p. 33–44.
9. Jarmon, L. Pedagogy, education and innovation in 3-d virtual worlds. Journal of Virtual Worlds Research 2009;2:(1). Available at: https://journals.tdl.org/jvwr/article/view/639/470. Accessed September 11, 2011.
10. Linden Lab. The Second Life homepage. Available at: http://secondlife.com/. Accessed September 15, 2011.
11. Linden Research, Inc. The Linden Lab homepage. Available at: http://lindenlab.com/. Accessed September 15, 2011.
12. SimTeach. Institutions and organizations in SL: universities, colleges & schools. Available at: http://www.simteach.com/wiki/index.php?title=Institutions_and_Organizations_in_SL#UNIVERSITIES.2C_COLLEGES_.26_SCHOOLS. Updated September 15, 2011. Accessed September 15, 2011.
13. Linden BK. Q1 2011 Linden dollar economy metrics up, users and usage unchanged. Available at: http://community.secondlife.com/t5/Featured-News/Q1-2011-Linden-Dollar-Economy-Metrics-Up-Users-and-Usage/ba-p/856693. Updated May 6, 2011. Accessed September 15, 2011.
14. Castronova E. Synthetic worlds: the business and culture of online games. Chicago: The University of Chicago Press; 2005.
15. Castronova E. Exodus to the virtual world: how online fun is changing reality. New York: Palgrave Macmillan; 2007.
16. Active Worlds, Inc. Active Worlds and education. Available at: http://www.activeworlds.com/edu/. Accessed September 15, 2011.
17. University of Texas at Arlington College of Nursing. Genomics translational research laboratory. Available at: http://www.uta.edu/nursing/genomics/. Accessed September 15, 2011.
18. University of Texas at Arlington in Second Life. Genomics journal club in Second Life. Available at: http://www.uta.edu/secondlife/genomicsjournalclub/. Accessed September 15, 2011.

19. Thompson D, Fisher A. Amputee Virtual Environment Support Space--a vision for virtual military amputee support. J Rehabil Res Dev 2010;47(6):vii–xii.

20. National Center for Telehealth & Technology.T2 virtual PTSD experience. Available at: http://t2health.org/vwproj/. Accessed September 15, 2011.

21. Yellowlees PM, Cook JN. Education about hallucinations using an internet virtual reality system: a qualitative study. Acad Psychiatry 2006;30:534–9.

22. Dunigan R. Vanderbilt University introduces new nursing technology. Available at: http://www.newschannel5.com/story/14293876/vanderbilt-introduces-new-nursing-technology. Updated March 22, 2011. Accessed September 15, 2011.

23. University of Texas at Arlington College of Nursing. The value of Second Life to nursing. Available at: http://www.uta.edu/secondlife/nursingce/. Updated November 6, 2011. Accessed September 15, 2011.

24. The Grid Live. The Far Away – a wheat field helping fight poverty. Available at: http://thegridlive.com/2007/12/28/the-far-away-a-wheat-field-helping-fight-poverty/. Updated December 28, 2007. Accessed September 15, 2011.

25. Linden Lab. Destination guide: Dublin. Available at: http://secondlife.com/destination/dublin. Accessed September 15, 2011.

26. Linden Lab. Destination guide: postgraduate medical school. Available at: http://secondlife.com/destination/postgraduate-medical-school. Accessed September 15, 2011.

27. Virtual Ability, Inc. Virtual Ability. Available at: http://www.virtualability.org. Accessed September 15, 2011.

28. Linden Lab. Educators – SL educators (The SLED list). Available at: https://lists.secondlife.com/cgi-bin/mailman/listinfo/educators. Accessed September 15, 2011.

29. Linden Lab. Healthcare – healthcare support and education. Available at: https://lists.secondlife.com/cgi-bin/mailman/listinfo/healthcare. Accessed September 15, 2011.

Immersive Virtual Reality Environments for Perioperative Nursing

Kelley Connor, MS, RN

KEYWORDS

• Virtual reality • Continuing education • Perioperative nurses

KEY POINTS

• Virtual reality environments offer the potential to expand professional development opportunities for perioperative nurses.

• Virtual reality education options include live interactive learning sessions for multiple users as well as self-directed learning for individual users.

• Examples of professional education opportunities in virtual reality include instructor-led simulations, lectures, group discussions, and poster sessions.

• Disadvantages to virtual reality education options include orienting the learner to the environment and the time involved by the educator to create and facilitate learning.

An overview of the Association for Operating Room Nurses Web site[1] reveals a robust online learning system in which registered nurses could access learning modules, continuing education articles and examinations, and both live and prerecorded Webinars. Although these offerings are numerous, immersive virtual reality (VR) environments may further expand opportunities for perioperative nursing education in an engaging and customizable format. Immersive VR environments utilize 3-dimensional online computer programs in which users interact with each other and the environment via touch, text, and voice through computerized representations of themselves called avatars.[2] Avatar appearance can be customized based on user preferences. Using a computer mouse, users can walk their avatar through the environment, touch objects, and interact with others. VR offers the potential for asynchronous learning where individuals can visit sites on their own similar to visiting a Web site to gain information. VR also offers the potential for synchronous learning. This is where individuals can meet online at a specific time and virtual space for the purposes of networking, group discussions, presentations, or simulation. This article

The author has nothing to disclose.
School of Nursing, Boise State University, 1910 University Drive, Boise, ID 83725-1840, USA
E-mail address: kelleyconnor@boisestate.edu

Perioperative Nursing Clinics 7 (2012) 251–255
doi:10.1016/j.cpen.2012.02.002
1556-7931/12/$ – see front matter © 2012 Elsevier Inc. All rights reserved.

describes the use of VR environments for perioperative nursing education and potential barriers to its use.

ADULT LEARNING THEORY

While VR is a relatively new educational tool, adult learning needs can be met based on adult learning theory principles. Knowles[3] characterizes adult learners as different from children as learners in that adults are capable of being self-directive, they have experiences to build on, and they have internal motivations for learning. For adult learners to best accept and learn new information, they must be able to see that new information is relevant to their needs. In addition, adult learners want to be able to see how they can immediately apply the new information.[3,4] Immersive VR is a good fit with the learning needs of adults, because the information can provide adults with the opportunity to learn relevant and applicable information in a variety of both synchronous and asynchronous formats.

VIRTUAL REALITY FOR INTERACTIVE LEARNING

Learning opportunities for perioperative nurses using immersive VR environments include group discussions, multimedia lectures, simulations, and tours through educational spaces. Several different VR options are available for educational use. Dalgarno and colleagues[5] surveyed the trend of 3-dimensional virtual world use in higher education and found 201 subjects offered in which 9% of respondents were health care educators. Further, 78% of these subjects were offered in *Second Life*. With more than 15 million registered members, *Second Life* is currently the most popular VR platform.[6] However, there are other platform options available, such as *Open Sim* and *Active Worlds*. Regardless of the platform, current trends indicate that VR is used in education for communication spaces, digital recreation of the physical environment, and for simulation experiences.[7]

Spaces and Communications

VR spaces offer the potential for asynchronous learning by self-directed or synchronous learning by faculty-directed tours of various sites. In a survey of health-related activities on *Second Life*, 34 of the 68 sites had a focus on education and awareness.[8] These sites included information presented on posters, bulletin boards, multimedia productions, slideshows, games, and links to Web pages. Topics varied and included sexual health, genetics, and environmental health hazards. Another example of a self-directed tour to learn a health concept is *Virtual Hallucinations*, where the experiences of people with schizophrenia have been recreated in VR.[2] Participants explore the environment while experiencing visual and auditory hallucinations. Researchers of the simulation surveyed participants who may or may not have been health care workers and found the majority of respondents believed the experience improved their ability to understand auditory and visual hallucinations, and 82% would recommend the experience to others.[2]

VR can be utilized as a communication space as a forum to conduct a synchronous meeting or lecture. These could be informal small group discussions, or an instructor may stand as an avatar on a virtual stage behind a podium and conduct a lecture while attendees sit in stadium style seats. I experienced this type of presentation example when I spoke at The University of Texas Arlington, College of Nursing in *Second Life*.[9] Speakers presented in a virtual outdoor auditorium and used Power-Point slides they advanced as needed. Attendees were invited to ask questions by text or voice. After the presentations, attendees could view poster presentations on display at the virtual exhibit hall. The benefit to this type of virtual presentation is that presenters and attendees were not limited by geography and could attend the offering from any location. Attendees were able to interact with the speakers, other attendees, and the virtual space around them, experiencing an environment similar to a live conference setting different from a Webinar or other online presentation.

Wiecha and coworkers[10] used this presentation method to study the effectiveness of conducting a 1-hour-long continuing medical education offering for primary care physicians using VR. The findings for this pilot study included an increase in pre- and posttest scores and an increase in confidence as reported by subjects, and all participants agreed that their learning session was effective. Furthermore, the respondents rated their *Second Life* experience as more beneficial than other online continuing medical education offerings and that they would recommend them to a colleague.

VR Simulation

Several examples of simulations have been developed for health care training in VR. VR simulations include scenarios in which learners interact in a realistic environment with their peers and an instructor. This section illustrates several examples of emergency cardiopulmonary response simulations, other simulation experiences, and mixed learning methods that include simulation conducted in VR.

In the first example, researchers conducted small group simulations of cardiopulmonary resuscitation (CPR) training. Students had to perform a series of CPR measures that included initiating treatment, relieving rescuers, and reporting to the oncoming paramedic and then repeat the VR scenarios after 6 months to evaluate learning decay.[11] Kilmon and coworkers[12] described a research project in which the team recreated the equipment, medications, and hospital environment used during a cardiac code. The objects and environment were programmed to respond to the actions of the user based on a touch screen monitor and Global Positioning Systems technology. The anticipated plan was that the team develops scenarios and a virtual patient to test their simulations with students and nurses. Bodily[13] has also developed emergency response equipment for CPR scenario training. In this case, the instructor controls the heart rate rhythms and the vital signs displayed on a cardiac monitor that is visible to simulation participants. The expected outcome is that participants are able to recognize the observed cardiac rhythm and intervene according to advanced cardiac life support standards.

In addition to cardiopulmonary resuscitation simulations, other VR simulations have been developed. Veltman and colleagues described a VR simulation based on a postpartum hemorrhage.[14] The students were to assess a patient and provide nursing interventions relevant to a hemorrhage, including lowering the head of the bed, obtaining vital signs, and providing fundal massage. Immediately after the simulation, a debriefing session was held with the students and faculty to reflect on the scenario. Phillips and Berge[15] provided an example of how VR was used in dentistry simulations in which the faculty logged on as avatar patients and students were to teach them about oral health.

Finally, there are sites that combine learning trends available in immersive VR by offering several different types of learning formats. One example that incorporates space for lecture format teaching, asynchronous self-directed learning, operating room simulations, and postanesthesia recovery simulations is located at Imperial College Islands.[16] Another example is the Allied Health & Science College, Munck,[17] where students have the opportunity to explore the environment and learn about radiopharmacy. In addition, educators are invited to participate in the experience by joining the site and offering their expertise.

Potential barriers

Potential barriers for perioperative nurses participating in continuing education include the inability to get time off from work, cost, and home responsibilities.[18] These barriers could potentially be overcome using VR as a delivery method. However, VR presents its own limitations. For example, VR offerings can often be labor intensive to create by the educators,[14] thus potentially limiting the amount of experiences available. Orientation to the VR environment could be a barrier for nurses seeking educational opportunities. It is important for the learner to be well oriented to the environment so the focus can be on the learning not the technology.[19] Other potential barriers include the need for reliable Internet connection, adequate Internet speed, and computers that meet the requirements for specific VR environments.

SUMMARY

Perioperative nurses require ongoing training and education to continually develop current evidence-based knowledge and skills. VR may be one of the ways nurses are able to acquire new information. VR offers the potential to increase the learning opportunities developed for and offered to perioperative nurses. Opportunities include small group discussions, large group classes, tours of educational sites, and simulations. Barriers for the learner to access VR education offerings include the computer requirements, Internet access, and orientation to the specific virtual environments. There are examples of VR used in health care education, and although not all of them are specifically geared to perioperative nurses' learning needs, they could be used as templates to be adapted for use with perioperative nurses in the future.

REFERENCES

1. AORN Web site. Available at: http://www.aorn.org/. Accessed November 6, 2011.
2. Yellowlees PM, Cook JN. Education about hallucinations using an internet virtual reality system: a qualitative study. Acad Psychiatry 2006;30(6):534–9.
3. Knowles MS. Andragogy in action. San Francisco: Jossey-Bass; 1984.
4. Smith MK, Knowles M. Informal adult education, self-direction and andragogy. The Encyclopedia of Informal Education Web site. 2002. Available at: http://www.infed.org/thinkers/et-knowl.htm. Accessed November 6, 2011.
5. Dalgarno B, Lee MJW, Carlson L, et al. An Australian and New Zealand scoping study on the use of 3D immersive virtual worlds in higher education. Australasian Journal of Educational Technology 2011;27(1):1–15. Available at: http://www.ascilite.org.au/ajet27/dalgarno.html. Accessed November 6, 2011.
6. WebProNews staff. Second life still alive and kicking. WebProNews Web site. May, 2009. Available at: http://www.webpronews.com/2009/03/16/second-life-still-alive-and-kicking/. Accessed November 6, 2011.
7. Hew KF, Cheung WS. Use of three-dimensional (3-D) immersive virtual worlds in K-12 and higher education settings: a review of the research. Br J Educ Technol 2010; 41(1):33–55.
8. Beard L, Wilson K, Morra D, et al. A survey of health-related activities on Second Life. J Med Internet Res 2009;11(2):e17.
9. University of Texas Arlington College of Nursing Center for Continuing Nursing Education. The Value of SecondLife life to nursing. Web site November, 2010. Available at: http://www.uta.edu/secondlife/news/. Accessed November 28, 2011.

10. Wiecha J, Heyden R, Sternthal E, et al. Learning in a virtual world: experience with using Second Life for medical education. J Med Internet Res 2010;12(1):e1.
11. Creutzfeldt J, Hedman L, Medin C, et al. Exploring virtual worlds for scenario-based repeated team training of cardiopulmonary resuscitation in medical students. J Med Internet Res 2011;12(3):e38.
12. Kilmon CA, Brown L, Ghosh S, et al. Immersive virtual reality simulations in nursing education. Nurs Edu Perspect 2010;31(5):314–7.
13. Bodily D. BP_VS_display_V1.43. Land of the Long White Cloud. SecondLife site. Available at: http://slurl.com/secondlife/Landofthelongwhitecloud/114/105/28. Accessed November 28, 2011.
14. Veltman M, Connor K, Honey M, et al. Collaborative practice through simulations in a Multi User Virtual Environment (MUVE). CIN Comput Inform Nurs 2011;30(2):63–7.
15. Phillips J, Berge Z. Second life for dental education. J Dent Educ 2009;73(11): 1260–4.
16. Medical Media Lab. Imperial College Islands. SecondLife site. Available at: http://slurl.com/secondlife/Medical%20School/48/133/26. Accessed November 6, 2011.
17. Allied Health and Science College, Munck. Radiopharmacy. SecondLife site. Available at: http://slurl.com/secondlife/Munck/171/230/3. Accessed November 6, 2011.
18. Schweitzer DJ, Krassa TJ. Deterrents to nurses' participation in continuing professional development: an integrative literature review. J Contin Educ Nurs 2010;41(10): 441–7.
19. Honey M, Connor K, Veltman M, et al. Teaching with Second Life®: hemorrhage management as an example of a process for developing simulations for multiuser virtual environments. Clinical Simulation in Nursing 2012;8:e79–85.

Implementation of an Electronic Health Record in a Perioperative Setting

Joshua M. Hawkins, BSN, RN, CPN

KEYWORDS

- Perioperative • Implementation • Electronic health record • Meaningful use criteria
- Barriers

KEY POINTS

- Electronic health record implementation.
- Perioperative implementation challenges.
- Generational differences and communication strategies.
- Change management in a perioperative setting.
- Application of meaningful use criteria to a perioperative EHR.

Computers have found their way into virtually all aspects of our lives. Computing technology is changing the way that we work, live, and interact. Health care has not been immune to this change. Traditionally, hospitals have been slow to adopt fully functional electronic health records (EHRs). It is currently estimated that only about 2% of all hospitals have a fully deployed EHR.[1] In 2009, this reality moved the U.S. government to impart a legislative ruling known as The Health Information Technology for Economic and Clinical Health Act. As part of the larger American Investment and Recovery Act, it laid out an incentive plan for hospitals to deploy EHRs that achieve meaningful use. The incentive takes the form of Medicare reimbursements before 2015 and Medicare penalties after 2015.

Meaningful use comprises a wide range of requirements that facilities must employ if they expect to receive reimbursement under the plan. Although the selection of the product that will be utilized is up to the individual facility or health care system, the product must meet the standards for meaningful use for hospitals to receive the reimbursement. Clinical products that have the additional certification of meaningful use through the office of the National Coordinator for Health Information Technology

The author has nothing to disclose.
Clinical Health Record, Implementation and Optimization, Baylor Healthcare System, 2001 Bryan Street, Dallas, TX 75201, USA
E-mail address: Joshuaha@baylorhealth.edu

Perioperative Nursing Clinics 7 (2012) 257–266
doi:10.1016/j.cpen.2012.02.005
1556-7931/12/$ – see front matter © 2012 Elsevier Inc. All rights reserved.

Box 1
What is meaningful use?

- Computerized physician order entry (CPOE): A licensed user may enter and manage orders into the EHR per state and national law.
- Implement drug-to-drug interactions and drug allergy interaction checking.
- Maintain an active and up-to-date list of past and present diagnosis.
- Maintain an active medication list.
- Maintain an active allergy list.
- Record the following demographic identifiers: date of birth, race, preferred language, ethnicity, and gender.
- Record and chart vital signs including height, weight, blood pressure, body mass index (BMI) calculation and display, and plotting of growth charts (including BMI) for children 2–20 years of age.
- Record smoking status for patients age 13 years and older.
- Report ambulatory clinical quality measures to CMS, or in the case of Medicaid to the states.
- Implement one clinical decision support rule, along with the ability to document adherence to that rule.
- Provide patients with an electronic copy of their health information (including laboratory tests, pertinent results, and documentation) upon request.
- Provide clinical summaries for each office/hospital visit.

---

have the added benefit of assurance of meeting meaningful use requirements. **Box 1** provides a list of data elements related to meaningful use according to the Office of the Coordinator for Health Information Technology's Web site.[2] The deployment of meaningful use EHR's have profound implications for perioperative settings.

BARRIERS TO ADOPTION IN THE PERIOPERATIVE SETTING

Despite the obvious advantages of EHR use as well as the government mandates, there still remains a significant amount of anxiety among staff members (and administration) surrounding the move from paper to electronic processes.[3] The reasons for this anxiety are diverse and unique to each individual. Although each staff member can have his or her own unique fears regarding EHR usage, a number of commonalities appear to cut across all segments of the nursing population. In the perioperative setting, the unique fast paced and time-sensitive environment of a surgical area comes with its own specific set of challenges such as ease of use, system architecture, limited staff input, generational differences, and fear.

Ease of Use

Ease of use is defined simply as how easy (intuitive) a system is to use. It is important for functions such as maximizing a window, scrolling through screens, double clicking, and drag and drop to operate the same as they do in a Windows or Macintosh environment. For most modern EHRs this is the case. However, a number of products remain in use that are still based on a nongraphic user interface (GUI) design and rely on a substantial amount of typing in Disk Operating System (DOS)–based architecture. Even in a GUI-based system, there remains the potential for frustration with regard to free texting redundant information. Additionally, typing speeds vary significantly among age groups and experience levels.

A nurse in his or her 20s may be able to type at a speed of 50 words per minute or more, in large part due to standard primary school education in computerized word processing. In contrast, a senior nurse may have had little or no exposure to typing.

System architecture designed to minimize free texting is essential when considering user acceptance. Speeds in mouse clicking are significantly less varied than are typing speeds. As such, nurses tend to express a much greater sense of ease with systems that integrate the mouse over the use of free texting (typing) observations. In addition to the human components, free texting can hinder the querying of data for the purposes of retrospective quality control and improvement. The computer is unable to differentiate items placed in free text fields from other standard, non-free text observations. Thus, many of the great benefits of an EHR are lost.[4]

System Architecture

There are a variety of components within the system itself that can influence a perioperative nurse's opinion of an EHR. One of the most common of these is the reported frustration with logging on and accessing the system. In one study that examined a group of nurses on a medical–surgical unit, 100% of the 11 nurses surveyed expressed frustration at the time that it takes to log in and access the system.[5] This problem is commonplace in many applications and tends to be a global issue, rather than an isolated occurrence. This is due in large part to rapid clinical software advances, which tend to advance much more slowly than hardware. This reality forces clinical applications to continue to utilize legacy operating systems to avoid compatibility issues (A. Tyner, Clinical Field Support, Dallas, TX, personal communication, August 18, 2011). A legacy system is simply a system that is in operation even when a newer version of the system exists. Legacy operating systems face major losses associated with performance gains that occur with newer versions of the operating system.[6] For example, the latest version of Windows (Windows 7) offers substantial improvements in speed, interface, and ease of use over the older options.

There are steps that can be taken to decrease login times, which can be built into applications. For example, many modern applications have a *suspend* function that will effectively pause the perioperative nurse's documentation so that he or she can leave the documentation for another task. One drawback is that using the suspend function effectively locks the computer for any other user. To unsuspend the terminal, the original user who initiated the suspend function must enter his or her password to resume documentation. This can be a serious problem when computers are in short supply.

Web-based EHR applications can present a major issue with login time. Web-based EHR applications store the program on a central Web server, rather than being installed locally on the computer's hard drive. Web-based applications have a major advantage in that it is substantially easer to upgrade applications when they are stored on a central server. To access a Web-based clinical application, the user must click on a link to open up a compatible Web browser. The perioperative nurse must then select the application from the window that he or she wishes to use and then log into the application itself. One health care facility substantially decreased login time by creating a single icon that allowed nurses to bypass the first step in the process.

Staff Input Before Rollout

Staff input is perhaps one of the most challenging areas for leadership when planning for the rollout of an EHR system. Staff perioperative nurses may hold the preconceived notion that their opinion does not affect the reality of the system's arrival and widespread use. This can be a symptom of a greater issue with workplace culture at large, but it necessitates attention nonetheless. Nursing administration can assist with this process by selecting individuals whom others would describe as comfortable with technology and change.[7] By selecting members of staff who are already well thought of in the realm of technology, nursing leadership can enhance staff acceptance and ensure that as many staff as possible have input into the system design. Traditionally, many EHR products are preconfigured with little room for customizability. Moreover, many hospital entities do not have dedicated clinicians who have the technical expertise to understand the needs of frontline clinical staff. This trend has changed in recent years. New products on the market allow a wide range of customization for the user to meet their needs. Although this does lead to the increased need for support personnel, the end result is a system that still meets regulatory requirements but is also usable in a wide range of specialty areas.[8]

Generational Differences

Generational theory states that people born during certain periods are influenced by the political, spiritual, and social landscape to develop certain common characteristics that separate them from people of other periods. Although the time periods themselves are open to some interpretation, there are generally agreed upon time ranges that classify generations. The Baby Boomers (born 1946–1964) tend to be very loyal employees. They grew up during a time of economic prosperity and change in the country. They are known to be hardworking and view overtime as an obligation rather than an option.[9]

Generation X (Gen X, born 1965–1976) tends to be tech savvy, independent, and self-directed. They can also be somewhat cynical and mistrusting of authorities. Members of this generation grew up during a time of intense change in America and were expected to grow up more quickly, but remained adolescents longer than previous generations did.[9] Gen X individuals tend to want action and lose interest if words are not backed up by actions. While they tend to embrace self-governance, they also tend to prefer working independently, rather than in a team.

The Millennials, also referred to as Generation Y (Gen Y), were born between 1977 and 1997. This group of individuals represents the newest group of individuals in the workforce. More than any other generation that preceded it, Gen Y embraces diversity, globalism, and technology as a part of life. Millenials tend to enjoy working in cooperative teams, but also enjoy the independence and flexibility of an open work schedule. Similar to Baby Boomers, Millennials have a strong sense of civic duty and work to achieve the greater good.[9]

Implementation

Knowledge of generational differences can greatly enhance the implementation of an EHR system in the perioperative setting. Millennials are widely considered to be the most techno savvy of the generations. To the Millennials, the line between life and technology is nonexistent; technology is a part of life. Given the young age of this generation, lack of clinical experience can be a very real issue. Millennials may be the quickest group to pick up on navigation and utilization of the system, but the previous two generations (Baby Boomers and Gen X) may find this threatening. The strengths of the Millennials', combined with the clinical expertise of the Gen X'ers and Baby Boomers, provides an excellent opportunity to bridge the differences between the generations.

Millennial nurses make excellent super users, as they tend to have exceptional command of technology. Baby Boomers often express fear of causing a malfunction in the system with standard use.[7] As such, there is often a great deal of fear surrounding an EHR. Millennials can ameliorate these fears by providing troubleshooting and proper escalation when needed. Pairing a Gen Y super user with a struggling Baby Boomer can develop a sense of mutual respect between these two generations. The Gen Y members offer their technical expertise and comfort with technology, while the Baby Boomer and Gen X'ers offer their vast clinical experience. Millennials can be an excellent support for Baby Boomers and Gen X'ers who require some extra one-on-one assistance to facilitate comfort with the new workflow. Millennials are also invaluable at extolling the benefits of an EHR.

Nurses commonly express a fear that an EHR product will substantially slow their work down. This can be very frustrating for staff nurses who already feel that they have too little time to perform their basic duties. The Millennial can demonstrate the reductions in time that the EHR can provide, while acknowledging that the change is difficult. Working together in this manner can have the serendipitous effect of enhancing cross-generational respect.

FACILITATORS TO EHR USAGE IN A PERIOPERATIVE SETTING

The benefits of EHR usage are well known. Access to a longitudinal historical record, interoperability between multiple clinical applications, increases in patient safety, and quality reporting metrics are just a few of the demonstrated values of an EHR.[1,10] In addition, the EHR reduces (or eliminates) the paper chart. In the past, clinicians could access only one patient care record at a time. With an EHR, users now have the ability to simultaneously access patient care records. This means that multiple users can simultaneously document on a single patient record, thus improving flow of information.

Historical data retrieval is one aspect of EHRs that is of particular interest to perioperative clinicians. For instance, instead of having to rely on the patient to recall medication information on each individual admission to the perioperative area, the nurse can simply pull the information from the last visit into the latest admission documentation. The nurse would then simply review the medication list and change the information as needed.

Information technology has come a long way since the days of large computers that covered city blocks. As a society, we are now more connected than ever. Smart phones allow us to connect with a huge network of friends using nothing more than a few swipes of a finger. New telecommunications technologies allow for virtual meetings over high bandwith connections. Everywhere, technology is changing the way that we live, work, and communicate. Health care has also embraced this trend, and powerful computers are now the standard in most facilities across the country. Workstations on Wheels (WOWs) offer nurses a compact way to go from patient bay to patient bay accessing information as needed. Wireless barcode scanning technology serves as an additional patient identifier before medications are administered. These will continue to develop into smaller, more efficient, less expensive, and more user friendly devices.[11]

Although the equipment used in our daily lives has improved substantially, these improvements are meaningless if the software used with the machine is not functional, user friendly, and dependable. As with hardware, human-focused software design has become much more prominent in the last decade. Before the advent of the GUI, users had to rely on text-based entry, with little to no standardization of icons. Thus, computer expertise was limited to a very small number of individuals. With the widespread use of the GUI interface, nurses can now utilize the much more user friendly method of a point-and-click interface.

Nurses may not be aware of the fact that on any given day, hundreds of different computer applications must work together to translate information into meaningful data. In the past, older EHRs (known as legacy systems) were not designed with interoperability in mind. The newest generations of EHRs have a high degree of interoperability. Interoperability is the ability of an EHR to talk to various different applications and to receive and send data to those applications. This is achieved by means of a standardized communication protocol known as Health Level 7 (HL7). This communication protocol is used as a standard way to communicate patient information across systems. Not every EHR is HL7 compliant, however, and this feature should be discussed when selecting a product. Without these features enabled there stands to be a substantial loss of functionality that stand to impact end users. Some real-world issues include documentation duplication, loss of clinical data flow, delays in results retrievals, and redundant maintenance of multiple clinical applications.[12] This all equates to a decreased amount of time to care for the patient.

CHALLENGES TO EHR IMPLEMENTATION IN A PERIOPERATIVE SETTING

The perioperative setting is unique, as are the challenges faced when implementing an EHR in the setting. First, the emphasis on time is considerably higher than on a standard patient care floor. According to one frontline nurse,

> Time constraints are an issue. The perioperative workflow necessitates smooth streamlined processes. They work off the clock and the perception of the clinical health record making jobs faster is more obvious here. In addition, operating room staff are managing multiple pieces of machinery, procedures, physicians and often times multiple pieces of software and this creates a difficult workflow at best (A Culley, RN, CNOR, Dallas TX, personal communication, October 2011).

Owing to the wide variety of clinical applications used in many perioperative settings, interoperability can be a challenge. Perioperative nurses frequently must document in several systems to meet requirements. One frontline informatics nurse expressed this particular concern during her unit's implementation of a new EHR:

> I think the biggest challenge we felt was the lack of integration between the different software that was in use. This was always a battle because Centricity Perioperative Manager (CPM) has never interfaced with any other program, but it seemed much worse after implementation of the new EHR in our department. CPM requires documentation in all caps, username and password included. It does NOT require you to log in after a period of inactivity. The new system required a user to acknowledge a log out pop up warning to stay logged in. CPM could not recognize when the user had to go outside of the program to access the new EHR, which is caps sensitive. The caps lock issue seems a small problem, but when you are chasing a fresh post op patient out of the room to recovery and have to print your documentation before you go there is no time to fiddle with *why* your password is not being accepted. Often this increased the turnaround time between cases because we had to go to recovery with the patient, give report, return to the OR and work out the password issues, and then return to recovery with your paperwork. Multiple successive password failures would also lock you out of the system if you did not catch your caps lock quickly enough (H. Rider, RN-BSN, CNOR, Waxahachie TX, personal communication, October 2011).

In general, electronic documentation can pose an overwhelming amount of information to a busy perioperative nurse. This anxiety can be traced to nursing documentation standards and norms. In traditional nursing education, nursing students are taught that they should avoid leaving any blank spaces in documentation. However, in an EHR a vast amount of data points and observations are laid out to cover every single observable patient state. With the limits of paper documentation length removed, an electronic document can cover substantially more observations. A typical perioperative nurse may fall prey to the mindset that he or she may need to document on every single observation, even when they are not applicable to the patient. It is essential that nursing leaders assist nursing staff with understanding that blank observations do not show up when clinical documentation is examined during audits. Observations that are required for the clinician to document are typically clearly identified by the system itself as mandatory. By assuring nurses that they should document only what they observe, leaders can help perioperative nurses gain a sense of confidence with the EHR.

There are also technical limitations associated with implementation of an EHR in a perioperative setting. For instance, a type of technology known as a Medical Device Interface (MDI) has the capability to pull the patient's latest vital signs automatically into the EHR, thus eliminating the need for the nurse to transcribe the information from a device into a medical record. The EHR will pull this information from the latest set of vital signs taken from the patient's electronic vital signs monitor. However, for the technology to function, the patient must be *bedded*, that is, he or she must be assigned a location within the system. If this crucial step is not done, then the timesaving features of the MDI will not function. Bedding a patient may not be feasible in a unit that has a fairly quick turnaround time. Additional full-time equivalents (FTEs) to support a clinical support staff member may not be feasible for individual units and smaller facilities.

RAMPING UP FOR IMPLEMENTATION

Nursing leaders should expect that there will be complications in the implementation planning phase. Nurse leaders must arm themselves with knowledge gleaned from other facilities and health care systems that have undergone an EHR transition. The 12 to 18 months leading up to an implementation must be used to effectively plan a successful rollout of the EHR system.

One of the most important decisions that facility leadership can face is the type of system the facility will be using. If the facility is part of a larger system, the facility may be limited to only the approved products in which the system has invested. It is essential that leaders include perioperative nurses in the product selection process. Nurses make up 2.6 million American jobs, tperioperative nurses in the product selectionhe largest number in the health care workforce.[13] Regardless of the system, nurses manage an overwhelming majority of patient care documentation. As such, they are the primary stakeholders in selecting a product that enhances workflow, patient safety, and is useable. Picking a product that is ready to go out of the box can be tempting for leaders, but the ability to personalize sections of the documentation layout can be limited. This issue would apply particularly to a specialty setting. In addition, nursing leaders must be careful to select products that are appropriate for their facility. A small ambulatory surgery center with fewer than 50 procedures per week should not select a product that is designed for a facility with 500-plus procedures per week. The additional costs associated with implementation should be taken into consideration as well. Additional training time will be needed for all staff who will use the EHR in their daily practice.[14] Staff should also be involved in equipment selection activities. Budgetary constraints should be shared with clinical staff as something to take into account when selecting equipment. Ideally, this equipment could be trialed by health care providers during open house type events. Nurses could then utilize an evaluation survey tool created in software such as Survey Monkey to identify their personal preferences in an anonymous manner. Equipment should be selected based on staff preference, durability, cost, and length of life.

Closer to the actual implementation date, 3 to 6 months, is typically when staff training takes place. Training typically takes place in a non production (pretend) environment. A training environment typically contains all the same features as a production environment, but does not use real patients. The training environment can sometimes change as new issues are identified with the product build before the date of go live. Placing staff education in this timeframe can help manage this issue. Last-minute changes to the EHR are inevitable, but this can be managed effectively by providing a comprehensive and custom-tailored education plan. Classroom time can be enhanced by encouraging nursing staff to practice documentation processes before implementation. One particular method, known as *shadow charting*, involves real, paper-based patient data. The nurse uses the paper documentation as the source for the concurrent practice activity, which takes place in the EHR practice environment. The patient name and account number in a practice environment are not associated with a real patient. Super users typically emerge during the training process. Super users are nurses who are frequently described as tech savvy and are sought by peers as experts in computing. These nurses are invaluable, as they combine a high level of technical aptitude with real-world clinical experience. When possible, super user participation should be integrated into general staff education. One method of doing this is to require super users to function as instructors during full staff education. Staff members who are educated by super users are more likely to feel that their concerns are being addressed and that they are being taught by someone who understands their individual practice. Super users given an in-depth overview of EHR functionality can ensure that there are as few gaps as possible between the current and future state of documentation.[15]

IMPLEMENTATION

The first days of implementation can be very challenging. Staff and leaders typically spend months planning for a successful implementation. To ensure as positive an experience as possible, some important steps need to be taken. The super users will be the greatest asset in the perioperative unit. Ideally, super users will not take any patients in the first 2 weeks of implementation. Super users must be free to identify and escalate issues to supervisors and information system department personnel, and to follow specified protocols when identifying breaks in the system. In addition, they need to be able to work one-on-one with users who require more personal attention.

Super users should be easily identifiable. Suggestions for easy identification include badges or pins and lanyards with bold color and logos. Whatever visual identifier has been chosen, the colors should be bright and quick to catch the eye.

Discussions should be held with leadership as to the FTE requirements for super users, as these nurses will represent nonproductive hours. A clear escalation plan is needed if super users encounter issues that they cannot answer during the implementation. Super users are the first line of defense when users identify issues during the rollout phase of implementation of the EHR. If the facility has a centralized reporting team or application, the super user should report those issues that cannot be solved by the super user. The super user should be submitting technical support cases on behalf of the clinician, as this process itself can be very tedious for a busy perioperative nurse.

Staffing patterns need to be taken into account, as new users can expect an increase in the amount of time that it takes them to document patient care. This is most noticeable in the first 3 months after implementation, and users can expect an average of a 50% increase in the amount of documentation time.[16] It is crucial that this reality is communicated to nursing staff before implementation, as many clinicians are under the belief that an EHR will instantly make their job more efficient. This is simply not the case.

There are multiple reasons for the inherent slowdown in documentation time. Perhaps the main reason is only that an EHR represents an entirely new paradigm with regard to documentation. Additional reasons for increased documentation time include hardware support issues, password and security role issues, and equipment failure. To manage these anticipated problems effectively, it is critical that staffing patterns be adjusted in the first 2 to 4 weeks of implementation.

In the perioperative area, discussions should be held with surgeons to decrease the normal case load associated with this area. Although this proposition may not be well received by medical staff, it nonetheless will make the implementation much smoother. Typically, nurse-to-patient ratios must be decreased in the implementation scenario. Perioperative areas have some slight flexibility, as elective cases can be planned well in advance. Communication with patients is also important during the implementation timeframe. A script given to staff before the rollout for use with patients can help patients understand why things might be taking slightly longer than normal. The following script is an example of a prompt that nurses can use when they experience technical difficulties with the system:

> "I apologize that we're having a little trouble—(accessing your information; scheduling your appointment; etc) at the moment. We're working to resolve the issue as soon as possible. Thank you so much for your patience."[17]

Although this exact script may not be appropriate for every encounter, it represents a patient-centered approach to addressing the inevitable issues that users can expect during the early days of implementation. As a reminder, example scripts can be printed, laminated, and placed on a badge tag.

SUMMARY

Rolling out an EHR in a perioperative setting is challenging. An EHR implementation represents an enormous amount of change, which can be so great that it can cause a massive amount of resistance from stakeholders. Using the lessons learned from other facilities that have faced this problem before, leaders can take the steps needed to help staff manage the changes successfully. In the end, the most important thing to remember is that at its core, an EHR is about facilitating the flow of information between patient and clinician. Reminding staff of this reality is one of the keys to keeping attitudes positive.

REFERENCES

1. Conn J. Still low tech: EHR adoption rates remain low: study. Mod Healthc 2009; 39(13):8–9.
2. Core Measures for Eligible Professional's with FAQ. CMS meaningful use overview. Available at: http://www.cms.gov/EHRIncentivePrograms/30_Meaningful_Use.asp#BOOKMARK1. Accessed November 4, 2011.
3. Lee TT, Mills ME, Bausell B, et al. Two-stage evaluation of the impact of a nursing information system in Taiwan. Int J Med Inform 2008;77(10):698–707.

4. Mahon PY, Nickitas DM, Nokes KM. Faculty perceptions of student documentation skills during the transition from paper-based to electronic health records systems. J Nurs Educ 2010;49(11):615–21.
5. Whittaker AA, Aufdenkamp M, Tinley S. Barriers and facilitators to electronic documentation in a rural hospital. J Nurs Scholarsh 2009;41(3):293–300.
6. Donovan J. Blueprint for a digital revolution. Health Manag Technol 2005;26(11):26.
7. Huryk LA. Factors influencing nurses' attitudes towards healthcare information technology. J Nurs Manag 2010;18(5):606–12.
8. Hyun S, Gakken S, Douglas K, et al. Evidence-based staffing: potential roles for informatics. Nurs Econ 2008;26(3):151.
9. Hahn JA. Managing multiple generations: scenarios from the workplace. Nurs Forum 2011;46(3):119–27.
10. Waxman S. EHRs offer significant medicolegal benefits—and risks: thorough documentation remains vital to avoiding malpractice lawsuits. Urology Times 2010;38(7):36.
11. Lipschultz A. A clinical engineer's predictions: the future of medical technology. Biomed Instrumen Technol 2008;42:42–4.
12. Glaser J. Interoperability: the key to breaking down information silos in health care. Healthc Financ Manage 2011;65(11):44.
13. Statistics USBoL. Registered nurses—occupational outlook handbook. Available at: http://www.bls.gov/oco/ocos083.htm. Accessed January 12, 2012.
14. Swab J, Ciotti V. What to consider when purchasing an EHR system. Healthc Financ Manage 2010;64(5):38–41.
15. McIntire S, Clark T. Essential steps in super user education for ambulatory clinic nurses. Urol Nurs 2009;29(5):337–43.
16. Sassen EJ. Love, hate, or indifference: how nurses really feel about the electronic health record system. Comput Inform Nurs 2009;27(5):281–7.
17. McCarthy C. Staff tips and scripting for EHR go live. Available at: https://www.mybaylor.com/Modules/Desktop/DocManager/StreamDocument.aspx?docID=141196. Accessed January 13, 2012.

Cyber Culture and Intercultural Communication Teaching, Learning and Collaboration

Lana Rings, PhD

KEYWORDS

- Perioperative nursing • Distance learning • Virtual environments
- Cross cultural communication

KEY POINTS

- Virtual simulation training in distance learning can help perioperative registered nurses further develop their skills.
- Simulation training in education provides the experiential learning needed for successful nursing practice.
- Technological issues must be explored for a cyber world that is in flux.
- Nonverbal and verbal intercultural communication should be addressed as pertinent to distance learning and professional practice.
- The legal and ethical implications of using social networks such as *Second Life* for professional purposes must be addressed as well.

Perioperative nurses must understand what is going on all times in the operating room. Circulating perioperative nurses have to be competent in nursing skills, able to foresee and prevent accidents and problems from occurring, make sure the patient is getting the best care possible (in essence be a patient advocate), and comfort patients in a place that feels foreign to them. Working in communities composed of people from diverse cultural and linguistic backgrounds, they must also have good intercultural communication skills when interacting with both fellow professionals and patients. Nursing education and continuing professional development can and should address all these issues in a world grown small. Training in all of these areas can and should also be provided in distance learning education, because of the advantages of cyberspace for connecting geographically disparate populations, and because of technology's ability to provide simulation training for nurses.

The author has nothing to disclose.
College of Liberal Arts, Department of Modern Languages, The University of Texas at Arlington, 701 Planetarium Place, Arlington, TX 76019–0557, USA
E-mail address: rings@uta.edu

Perioperative Nursing Clinics 7 (2012) 267–282
doi:10.1016/j.cpen.2012.02.011
1556-7931/12/$ – see front matter © 2012 Elsevier Inc. All rights reserved.

For learners to take advantage of the benefits of learning in cyberspace, there are a number of factors affecting whether one is a "have" or "have-not" in the interconnected Web world. Whereas it is true that electronic communication is changing the way in which the health care and educational communities provide their services (witness the emergence of electronic medical records and distance learning, for example), yet not all populations have equal access. Internet connectivity is not equalized across the nation. In household use, "rural America lags behind urban areas by ten percentage points (60% vs 70%)."[1] Yet rural nurses, as well as nurses in large metropolitan areas, should be able to benefit from distance learning. There are efforts underway to provide funding to "bring high-speed Internet to the 6% of the population that has been saddled with slow or no Internet and is losing ground economically and academically as high-speed Internet have-nots."[2] Indeed the goal of the Obama administration is broadband access for 10 million rural Americans.[3]

Comfort and experience with the technological aspects of cyberspace, together with an understanding of online culture, also affect one's willingness to access the potential of distance education. Those who are comfortable with the technology will not have the emotional drag that they otherwise would have, and gaining experience with the technology provides a better attitude toward it.[4] As the younger generations grow older, it is quite possible that the comfort level will shift in the populations in cyberspace.

Furthermore, from knowing abbreviations and texting shortcuts to Internet etiquette, or netiquette, of various kinds in virtual reality, there is an enculturation period. Thus, emoticons like the smiley face are icons that express specific intentions of the user, as well as emotional and nonemotional meanings.[5] Different languages and cultures differ in their use and interpretation of the Internet.[6,7]

As access becomes ever more possible, the potential benefits of simulation training in cyberspace can be far-reaching for otherwise geographically unreachable learner populations who need to further their professional development. Learning in virtual environments (VEs) can serve in-servicing types of functions and address annual reiterations of knowledge. Research already demonstrates the efficacy of simulation training with repetitive practice in virtual reality, because it is being used and tested in fields as distinct as medical training and the military. Surgeons, for example, are able to hone their skills in laparoscopic surgery through virtual simulation training[8] and in the military, practicing space maneuvers in virtual three-dimensional (3D) worlds is possible as well.[9] Furthermore, professional education is encouraging such types of learning; a number of universities are already using 3D worlds in nursing education and a few are trying it out in distance learning contexts.[10]

As in on-campus simulation in smart hospitals,[11] virtual simulation training is an excellent form of experiential learning, providing experiences very similar to face-to-face simulation.[8] Skill development, problem-solving, intercultural communication, and collaborative team work, all benefit from virtual simulation training, and such learning, because it is experiential, can be transformative.[12]

Additionally, students who feel safer hiding behind their computer screen can possibly express themselves and be heard more comfortably, or those who are tongue-tied in the classroom can write deeper analyses of what they are learning, if called on to do so.[13] Finally, and importantly, the impact on patients can be significant, because they can be secure in the knowledge that their health care providers have been through such thorough and repetitive real-world training.

Today's world challenges for continuing skill development and education, however, are twofold: technological and intercultural. First, in perioperative nursing education the environment that must be simulated virtually is the operating room (OR), and therefore the following physical layouts and interactive constraints must be taken into consideration: In the OR professionals work across a table from each other, wearing masks and communicating through subtle hand gestures, eye contact, and body language, and often with colleagues from different backgrounds. At all times they must interpret the flow of events and be able to act spontaneously in crisis situations, working seamlessly in collaboration with others. Circulating registered nurses (RNs), as patient advocates in the OR, must be attentive and vigilant, compensating because neither focused surgeon nor anesthetized patient can, for example, react to a patient's leg that has fallen off the table. RNs must also communicate with patients, sometimes using touch and eye contact while respecting culture-specific rules for linguistic and nonverbal behavior. Furthermore, they are to create bonds of connection, trust, and a sense of safety for the patient who is in the foreign world of the OR. Technology must provide the simulation environments in 3D virtual worlds in which such interactions can be practiced.

Second, sophisticated understanding of intercultural communication is also needed, in both distance and face-to-face learning as well as in the workplace itself, because students, educators, medical professionals, and patients come from a variety of backgrounds, cultures, and languages. From large population centers to small rural communities, hospital personnel represent a diversity of cultures. Even in a small rural hospital a patient may have an African American RN, an Anglo-American surgical technologist, a primary physician from India, and an anesthesiologist from Southeast Asia. Student, educator, and patient populations are just as diverse. In the Dallas, Texas, Independent School District, for example, 60 languages are spoken in households within the district,[14] and in Oregon, 11.7% of the population is now Hispanic.[15] Immigrants continue to come, now "primarily from Asia and Latin America, a trend expected to intensify in the 21st century."[16] Thus, one can encounter Euro-American, Mexican American, and Asian American cashiers and baggers in small-town America.

The following two examples from simulation training in a distance-learning course illustrate the convergence of the technological and the cultural challenges in cyberspace, where educator and student experience with the tools is often still relatively new. It should first be noted that a 3D virtual world is akin to a video game, with scenes and settings projected to represent reality. Animated figures called avatars, "computer-generated visual images" or "synthetic characters. . .for computer users,"[17,18] are operated by a human controller. However, unlike video game contexts, virtual worlds are used to "create simulated experiences" for nongaming purposes.[19]

An educator must train students to use the technology specific to the virtual environment he or she is using. In the VE *Second Life*, students must learn, for example, how to obtain virtual professional clothing for their avatars. One educator did not realize that when she made a certain move for her avatar to change clothes, her avatar became undressed in front of the other avatars, in other words, her students. Although she was in reality physically clothed, she nevertheless experienced a feeling of embarrassment. If avatars are an extension of the self, as some say they are, and since nudity is unacceptable for both educator and nurse, it is no wonder that she felt naked emotionally. In another instance, she could not get her cursor to work properly, and her avatar kept bumping into another avatar on the screen (J.D. Baker, Arlington, TX, personal communication, January 27, 2012).

In addressing technological problems while using an avatar, one must decide the proper behavioral response. In the scenario described previously, apologizing would be appropriate in the US culture in physical reality, but the repetition of the act becomes a response to a technological problem that participants come to recognize. When then does one stop saying "excuse me" or "I'm sorry" and address the bumping as an aspect of user interface problems? Furthermore, cultural interpretations come into play as well. If, for example, one is a member of a culture where one does not necessarily apologize for bumping into another unless one inconveniences the other in a major way, the false interpretation of different cultural rules can lead to misunderstanding and negative feelings among the participants. Thus, the interactive issues that may arise within the virtual space can compound the complexity of the situation.

Ultimately, intercultural communication skills are critically important to nursing professionals when interacting with patients and fellow health care professionals. In distance learning through simulation, however, multiple layers of interaction allow for intercultural communication problems to occur, as well as provide an opportunity to address them and to gain additional needed skills in our multicultural world.

Whereas it has now been well-understood for a number of years that that competence in cross-cultural interactions is critical to successfully extending health care to all,[20] this article expands on that discussion by exploring the importance of intercultural communication skills in general, and of simulation learning in cyberspace in particular. It also takes up the discussion of the use of 3D virtual worlds in perioperative nursing distance learning. The next section addresses critical issues in intercultural communication in some depth. A discussion of the technological benefits and challenges of simulated distance learning in 3D virtual worlds follows.

INTERCULTURAL COMMUNICATION SKILLS AT THE CONCEPTUAL, WORD, PHRASE, AND TEXTUAL LEVELS

To be able to successfully communicate with people who are different, in rank, background, experience, ethnicity, culture, and/or language, a specific form of cultural sensitivity and intercultural communication skill is needed. Successful relationships must be based on mutual trust, respect, and understanding, and on giving the other the benefit of the doubt. Intercultural communication education can go a long way to help professionals develop genuine tolerance, so that they can more readily attain their goals to help patients. A working definition of culture provides the basis on which to explore intercultural nonverbal and verbal behavior. Culture is composed of "the values, symbols, interpretations, and perspectives that distinguish one people from another.. . . People in a culture usually interpret the meanings of symbols, artifacts, and behaviors in the same or in similar ways."[21]

People from different cultures, however, often tend to interpret the symbols, artifacts, and behaviors, both nonverbal and verbal, differently from one another and in culturally specific ways. Broad concepts and behaviors that are culturally determined include the use of time and space, the concept of individualism and community, equality, the avoidance of uncertainty, indulgence, short-term orientation, and the "gendering" of human males and females (the expectations regarding talk, dress, behavior, and interaction).[22]

Whereas differences exist between individuals within a culture, nevertheless cultural groups tend to share many of the same interpretations, and speakers tend to interpret language in quite culture-specific ways. Unfortunately, when cultures collide, misunderstanding occurs, and the differences are not perceived as such, but rather as indications of spiteful intentions, rudeness, an uncooperative attitude, or severe character flaws on the part of the other. Both nonverbal and verbal communication behaviors play a role in the way human beings shape their culture-specific conceptions of reality.

Nonverbal Behavior

Scholarship in health care recognizes the importance of cross-cultural differences in nonverbal behavior.[23,24] Whether face-to-face or in cyberspace, awareness is the first step in appropriate response and understanding cross-cultural interaction. Campinha-Bacote[25] proposes a model of competent health care delivery based on the following assumptions about cultural competence:

1. Cultural competence is a process, not an event.
2. Cultural competence consists of five constructs: cultural awareness, cultural knowledge, cultural skill, cultural encounters, and cultural desire [described as the desire to understand another group].
3. There is more variation within ethnic groups than across ethnic groups (intra-ethnic variation).
4. There is a direct relationship between the level of competence of health care providers and their ability to provide culturally responsive health care services.
5. Cultural competence is an essential component in rendering effective and culturally responsive services to culturally and ethnically diverse clients.[25]

Cross-cultural competence is also important in simulation scenarios, because avatars interact and react nonverbally in many of the same ways that the humans controlling them do. Whether in cyberspace or physical space, people tend to use their culture-specific ways of behaving and moving,[26] and avatars are coming to be perceived as extensions of the human beings who control them. Real-time human-to-avatar motion capture is being developed so that anything the human does, his or her avatar is able to do.[27] Indeed, there are those who maintain one should be held legally accountable for one's avatar's behavior and any emotional or financial damage that it may cause.[26]

Much communication is nonverbal and is therefore an important aspect of human interaction, even in cyberspace. Several aspects of nonverbal behavior that are important for 3D worlds are summarized in the following discussion: the use of space (proxemics), eye movement (oculesics), specifically eye contact, touch (haptics), movement (kinesics), and laughter.

Proxemics addresses the "perception and use of space."[28] When meeting face-to-face, for example, those from cultures where one is expected to stand within about 12 inches of another's face will be constantly attempting to move toward someone who normally stands 2 feet or more away from one's conversation partner.[29] Both will be irritated, and both will misinterpret the behavior: as insult or brashness. Furthermore, in some cultures one stands closer in line (middle-class German), when compared with other cultures (middle-class US American).[30] When the unaware Germans cut in, according to the American, they are called rude. Yet, they do not see that the American is standing in line (P. Nest, personal communication, April 26, 1993). Similarly, research shows that avatars are placed next to others' avatars in similar ways that humans place themselves in physical reality. If two avatars isolate themselves, that behavior is interpreted as it would be in face-to-face situations.[26] It follows that cross-cultural space issues can surface even between avatars.

Eye movement (oculesics) is also interpreted differently depending on one's cultural background. In the United States one values looking another in the eye, because it expresses one's trustworthiness and forthrightness.[31] In the Korean culture, on the other hand, if one is a subordinate, he or she is expected to divert his or her gaze unless answering a superior's questions.[32] Avatar gaze, too, affects the interaction. Avatars whose gaze seems focused in natural ways, as opposed to those with random gaze, are interpreted as more effective.[33] Because gaze is possible with avatars, it will be interpreted in culture-specific ways as well.

Furthermore, knowledge of whom one may touch and how often is also culture-specific. In some cultures people touch frequently, whereas in others, they do not. Touch is dependent on roles. A higher ranked person may often touch a lower ranked person, whereas the opposite is not the case.[34] Again, an avatar bumping into another avatar will be interpreted as if the human controller were bumping into the other human.[26]

Finally, the meaning of laughter also varies. In the Japanese culture, laughter provides other interactional signals besides joy: identification with one's in-group, easing tension, evasion and the avoidance of saying something uncomfortable, masking embarrassment, or bewilderment.[35] Hearing laughter in cyberspace will be interpreted according to one's culturally based expectations of the appropriateness of laughter in the situation.

If educators and students, nurses, practitioners, or patients are unaware of the potential for miscommunication, some will be offended and will work more reluctantly with, or with less trust of, the other.[16] Indeed, how a nurse touches a patient, for example, will be interpreted by that patient as positive or negative, reassuring or invasive. This tendency is equally true in cyberspace. In the future, it will be even more so, as real-time human-to-avatar motion capture becomes common in more environments.[27]

Language and Meaning

If the nonverbal world is complex, so too is the world of language, perhaps more so. It is not much of an exaggeration to say that any word that comes out of our mouths is culturally bound, has culture-specific meanings, and is therefore ripe for misinterpretation when people from different backgrounds interact. In fact, Wierzbicka[36] maintains that there are but a few words, perhaps 36, that are completely and totally universal in their meaning. The acquisition of a native language thus implies the acquisition of the native, culture-specific meanings humans accumulate, over years of hearing and using words in specific context. They are heard and used within the family, neighborhood, school, church, workplace, social groups, and other parts of the community, to describe particular objects, events, situations, abstractions, or feelings, or to accomplish specific goals (impressing, persuading, informing, showing friendliness, and so forth). Beginning at the word level and proceeding to ever longer linguistic utterances, the discussion that follows highlights how fragile communicating across cultures can be. Students and educators from different cultures will have to be aware of the possibilities for mistaken understanding, especially when they cannot see each other and when their avatars are playing different roles for them.

Words such as *house, hospital,* and *anger* hide meanings that people from differing backgrounds assume when using those words. Take, for example, the word *house.* The more different the cultures and backgrounds of the partners in a conversation, the more different the image one conjures up when hearing the word *house.* However, it is not just the size or the structural design, the materials of which it is made, and house color that reside in that meaning. It is also the space around it, the neighborhood one expects, as well as which people may inhabit it (nuclear family, multigenerational family, family and nonfamily members). In addition, what goes on inside of it is also embedded in the concept of *house*: lots of gatherings or few gatherings, meals together or separate, studying at the kitchen table or in a bedroom or study. But it does not stop there. The meanings change depending on the context. Consider the difference between *the houses in my hometown* and *the newer houses on the block in the new subdivision*. One must know what a hometown or a subdivision entails, and in what era they exist(ed). Finally, the emotions play a role in one's definition: whether one looks on particular kinds of houses favorably or not depends on what kinds of emotional experiences one has surrounding them. A particular house resembling the one in which the family dynamics were painful may bring back distressing memories.

Words denoting emotions are also culture-specific. Whereas all human beings have emotions, nevertheless words describing emotions can be culture-specific. Wierzbicka[36] maintains that the word *anger* is not universal in all its nuances, although many think that it is. She says:

> The way people interpret their own emotions depends, to some extent at least, on the lexical [vocabulary] grid provided by their native language. Two different creatures (eg, a large nocturnal moth attracted by lights and a clothes moth) may be classified as "the same kind of creature" (in English) and as "two different kinds of creature" in Polish. . .. The same applies to emotions: whether or not two feelings are interpreted as two different instances of, essentially, "the same emotion" or as instances of "two different emotions" depends largely on the languages through the prism of which these emotions are interpreted.[36]

Words also express culture-specific values. For example, a key Anglo value is being reasonable, and its attitudes are expressed in *it is reasonable to*, *reasonable doubt*, *reasonable care*, *a reasonable time*, and *reasonably good*:

> A few hundred yards from my home there is a preschool, with a sign warning that "any person who trespasses on these premises without a reasonable excuse may be prosecuted." Every time I pass this school, I am struck by how Anglo and how untranslatable its phrasing is, with its reliance on the key Anglo concept "reasonable" – untranslatable into my native Polish, into French, German, and, I believe, any other language of the world.[37]

Single words also can represent important cultural institutions, as well as vast areas of knowledge and experience shared by the members of one culture. The terms *health care*, *disease*, *nudity*, *touch*, *religion*, and *government* and their interrelationships represent a multitude of experiences and meanings. Analogous to the situation with *house*, one's understanding and interpretation of the words *disease* and *health care* vary depending on one's experiences, and the greater the differences in cultural definitions of disease and their treatment, the greater the misunderstandings that can occur when people from different cultural backgrounds discuss them.[38]

> "Disease" is an elusive entity. It is not simply a less than optimum physiological state. The reality is obviously a good deal more complex; disease is at once a biological event, a generation-specific repertoire of verbal constructs reflecting medicine's intellectual and institutional history, an occasion of and potential legitimation for public policy, an aspect of social role and individual – interpsychic – identity, a sanction for cultural values, and a structuring element in doctor and patient interactions. In some ways disease does not exist until we have agreed that it does, by perceiving, naming, and responding to it.[38]

Thus, the definition of disease, its causes, what should be done about it and when, where, how, and by whom, as well as other cultural concepts like religious beliefs and political policy that may affect it, all come to bear on the understanding of the word.

Locution, Illocution, and Perlocution

Single words are only the tip of the intercultural communication iceberg, however, and situations and context begin to determine more culture-specific meanings of words and their uses. As is the case with nonverbal communication, people can completely misunderstand each other without knowing they are doing so. Speech act theory[39] explains this possibility well. According to a simplified, but usable, definition of this theory, there are three levels of understanding that occur when one person speaks to another. The first, called the locution, is an understanding of the words, as in, "Hi, how are you?" Native and nonnative speakers of a language usually understand all four words, for each is a high-frequency word. The second level is the speaker's interpretation of the words, or the illocution. Here the context of situation comes into play. The native speaker of American English may be a cashier in a grocery store in certain parts of the United States. For her, "Hi, how are you?" is a polite greeting and conversational opener for the service encounter that she is beginning with the next customer in line. In this situation, she does not think of its other possible meaning, in other words, an expression of concern about the physical, mental, or emotional well-being of another.

The third level of understanding, called the perlocution, is the listener's interpretation of the message, again within the context of the situation. A young male, a native speaker of German, having just arrived in the United States to be an au pair, or nanny, for an American-German couple, has been asked to go to the grocery store and pick up some items. In the German culture, "Hi, how are you?" is not used in service encounters with strangers, but rather with people one knows and with whom one has some sort of relationship. At a German supermarket, "Hello," "Good morning," or "Good day" is used as a greeting. Thus, the young man misinterprets the young woman cashier's greeting as interest in him. ("Why else would she say that?" he thinks. Since they are both young, maybe she is interested in him.) It does not cross his mind that "Hi, how are you?" might serve as no more than a friendly greeting and service encounter opening. He answers with the following: "Well, I have had this root canal problem. . . ." He stops at that point, because he sees the look of consternation on her face. He is confused. In this actual event, her reaction was one of perplexity and his was disappointment that "Americans don't really say what they mean."[40]

In the reverse situation, an American in Germany might think "good day" seems more stilted than what he or she considers a normal greeting. In fact, many commonly used phrases, such as good-byes, requests, invitations, apologies, warnings, and compliments are all examples of speech acts that may differ in meaning, connotation, and use from one language and culture to another, or even within subcultures.

Conversations

However, misunderstanding does not stop there. Conversational structure, including how one structures arguments, provides problems as well. In particular situations in Chinese or other Asian cultures, for example, the main point, comment, or action suggested in a conversation occurs after the background information or reasons for them are stated, whereas the opposite is true for most Western speakers of English, who expect the main point first, then the reasons afterwards. Thus, a Chinese person will say:

> Because most of our production is done in China now, and uh, it's not really certain how the government will react in the run-up to 1997, and since I think a certain amount of caution in committing to TV advertisement is necessary because of

the expense. So, I suggest that we delay making our decision until after Legco makes its decision.[41]

But someone with a more western orientation might say:

I suggest that we delay making our decision until after Legco makes its decision. That's because I think a certain amount of caution in committing to TV advertisement is necessary because of the expense. In addition to that, most of our production is done in China now, and it's not really certain how the government will react in the run-up to 1997.[41]

(The first example is from an actual conversation. The second was created by the authors. It is for this reason that one sees the "uh's" and nonsentential syntax in the Chinese utterances, but not in the Western rendition of the ideas. They are not due to the Chinese speaker's lack of linguistic skill.)

These two examples demonstrate why there might be some confusion when representatives from the two different traditions attempt to work together. Thus "arise the unfair and prejudicial stereotypes of the 'inscrutable' Asian or of the frank and rude westerner."[41] Again, there is misunderstanding, because of the differences in the illocution (speaker's interpretations) and the perlocution (listener's interpretations), and neither interlocutor is aware of it.

Even within the Western tradition, differences exist between cultures. Germans and Swiss speakers will tend toward similar strategies in conversations, whereas US American and British speakers will tend toward others. In many German environments, it is important to address deep issues about politics and controversial issues to get to know someone or to interact with guests in one's home. In addition, heated debates are considered fun and enjoyable. Conversely, in many similar US American environments it is important to address commonalities when getting to know others or staying in their home. One does not normally begin by arguing in these situations or debating about politics. The resulting interpretations of the conversations are that the Germans are rude, according to many Americans, whereas the German speakers think the Americans are superficial.[42] Similar discourse strategies ring true in Swiss-British conversations as well.[43]

Within conversations themselves, rules exist as to when and how conversation partners can overlap (negatively viewed as interruption) and how people can hold the floor and continue talking. French and New York speakers tend to overlap more in conversations than other middle-class US American speakers. Thus, they are found to be rude in cases when, according to their cultural definitions, they actually are contributing interest, help, and good manners to the conversation. They, in turn, tend to find those who wait for an opening rather dull or unhelpful in carrying the conversation along.[44,45]

Such ways of talking vary within a culture and, of course, across cultures. Certain groups within a culture may be allowed to speak less often, in specific situations, than they would in other cultures. Similarly, those cultures with more overlap, too, will tend to dominate the conversation when engaged with those with less overlap, with the resulting negative reactions.

All of these linguistic behaviors point to the fact that human beings have a kind of script in our heads regarding how nonverbal and verbal interactions should occur.[46] They demonstrate that if participants deviate from what is expected in the script, then it causes the listeners or readers to think about their interpretations of those deviations. When those deviations come from people from different backgrounds, one does not tend to attribute their behavior to their culture-specific upbringing or to their cultural norms, but rather to their ("terrible") personalities.

Therefore, whole texts, whether conversations, as those discussed previously, or long texts like books, can be interpreted very differently across cultures. Salman Rusdie's *Satanic Verses*, for example, is a case in point. Many members of the Muslim world thought it was too irreverent, whereas other people took no offence.[47]

Power and Rank

Finally, power and rank issues can exist within hospitals, and the urgency of the OR provides possibilities for the increase in tensions in interaction.[48,49] In settings where nurses and doctors are from different backgrounds, languages, cultures, and countries, this problem can be exacerbated. The perceived formality between nurses and doctors and the status of nurses and doctors within the community socializes them to specific language behaviors and uses. Beliefs about the ways nurses, physicians, and technologists should interact with each other and with patients come into play in cross-cultural settings. The need for better understanding is evident for a just culture in which an understanding of all the above exists and in which the benefit of the doubt, mutual respect, and trust are nurtured.

Cyberspace is similarly complex. Avatars change roles in a simulation environment (from students and educator to various nursing personnel and physicians). Indeed, in the cyber world there are three layers of social interaction and potentially of status issues. The first comprises the computer users themselves and their relationship to each other. Second, the avatars' relationships with each other are based on those of their controllers (although technological skill will often give one a more dominant role).[50] Third, in addition to representing their controllers (students and educators), the avatars represent the roles that they play (as health care professionals). As extensions of the learners and educators, they will speak in ways that are culturally appropriate to their human controllers, given the specific situation at hand. Thus, their ways of talking in cyberspace will be constrained by their role relationships and by their cultural influences.

Given all these possibilities for misunderstanding, the most grave issue involved in cross-cultural misunderstanding and miscommunication is the fact that very often people do not know that they are misunderstanding or being misunderstood. In most of the instances provided here, the intentions of the speakers and listeners were falsely interpreted by the others without their knowing it. They were basing their interpretation of the other's behavior on their own cultural rules, and they thought that they were communicating clearly. Every patient encounter by the perioperative RN has the same potential communication issues.

CYBERSPACE FOR PERIOPERATIVE EDUCATION: OPPORTUNITIES AND CHALLENGES

Intercultural issues are one aspect of distance learning in simulation scenarios in cyberspace, with implications for the OR. Simulation technology also presents opportunities and challenges that frame the way in which teaching and learning occur in collaborative spaces.

As stated earlier, nursing skills can be learned and honed through repetitive practice in simulation exercises in virtual environments. This potential is true not only for commonly occurring situations in the OR, but also for the simulation of low frequency and high-risk events. Although the perioperative RN may or may not encounter these events within the lifetime of a career, repetitive practice with such scenarios fosters critical skills that will be needed: the ability to successfully respond to a health care problem seen for the first time by interpreting it appropriately and determining the kinds of precautions that are needed. It also provides repetitive opportunities to work, interact, and communicate with others toward flawless team performance. Sample scenarios include low frequency pediatric scenarios, disaster planning and implementation, and hyperthermia events. In the latter case, in which an infrequently occurring but life-threatening problem is encountered, RN students must decide what to do as the patient's temperature radically drops. Finally, for testing purposes, similar scenarios can then be presented as problems to be solved. From a practical point of view, a wise allocation of time and concentration is needed to address the skills renewal, new skills development, and high-risk, infrequent event simulation that professionals need.

Skilled information technology (IT) specialists are needed to help create, in collaboration with faculty (through academic or staff development), scenarios that meet these needs. These personnel are critical in developing such mundane items as clothing for avatars (scrubs, uniforms, patient gowns, and so forth), as well as special aspects of the operating room. Potentially, they will be responsible for developing programmed recognition of such physical phenomena as the sensations of water while washing hands or a patient's pain response. For example, if a nurse reaches up to start an intravenous procedure without proper protocol and is accidentally pulling on a patient's arm, thus causing pain, then the patient might cry out in pain. These types of illustrations must be created in the environment for the simulation to work and seem like the real situation.

Such design costs money, in terms of purchasing design time and expertise and reducing faculty workloads in one area to compensate for the other. Furthermore, a virtual environment like *Second Life*, which is a proprietary product, charges if one wishes to build up assets within it. Whereas the *Second Life* software that one has to download is free, nevertheless one must purchase space to create within the environment.

There are additional challenges as well. Universities and health care facilities must be willing to support such activities. They are more likely to support endeavors that reach a critical mass of students and fulfill a critical societal need. However, if there is risk of losing significantly, for example if for some reason the technology proves too expensive and the venture fails or if it is not cost-effective, then universities or health care facilities will be cautious about their support. Furthermore, if the virtual environment being used is superseded by a new format, causing IT design to shift away from the current one, the question will be whether and how one can convert it and how expensive it is to do so. One need only recall how VHS (Video Home System) replaced the allegedly superior Betamax format in the 1980s.

Third, there are issues related to intellectual property, especially defining public versus private (student and educator) rights to the work done in virtual environments. Other questions include: How does one protect student/patient privacy while disseminating information to the public that is critical to its needs? If one has built a virtual environment like an operating room in *Second Life*, does one have the right to place it in a different VE platform? What rights does the vendor have? In addition, how much protection of one's content is there in this cyberspace environment?[51,52]

Finally, *Second Life* is a social networking site. As in all social networking, one must navigate the personal, social, professional, and legal ramifications of behavior in this space, even by one's avatar. Unfortunately, the line of demarcation is not clear and raises a number of concerns: How does one keep one's professional and personal life separate? What should be done if students do not wish to use their private avatar personas for their student or professional avatars? Should the professional avatar persona look different from the way it does in social use? Furthermore, how much professional distance does the site allow, and how can/should one establish parameters? Should a nursing educator friend a student in *Facebook* and vice versa? Should a nurse friend a patient in *Facebook*? What are the legal, ethical, and moral ramifications of such behavior? What is the responsible thing to do? Which tools are appropriate for which sites? Social networking platforms tend to blur cyber relationships.

As students become more professional, they tend to use social networks like *Facebook* less; however, unprofessional use in the early stages of medical education has been documented.[53,54] Therefore, educating students about "e-professionalism" is warranted, to include "how online personas may blend into professional life; and . . . the risks of online social networking."[55]

AWARENESS AND BEHAVIOR: ADDRESSING CROSS-CULTURAL COMMUNICATION SUCCESSFULLY

The questions discussed here raise a number of issues, bringing us full circle to the ways in which human beings interact within and across cultures to get our needs met, to live life the way we wish to, to further our careers, and to help those in need and those about whom we care. In cyberspace, as well as "on the ground," in addition to pure knowledge and nursing skills practice, intercultural communication training is, can, and should be an integral and necessary aspect of nursing education. Thus, a few words are appropriate concerning awareness and techniques to use in addressing intercultural communication, and communication in general.

Even if speaking the same language, it is important to remember that knowing the same words does not necessarily translate into having the same meanings for those words. Remembering that language is culturally loaded will help a person to slow down and take stock of a situation. If the emotions of frustration or anger surface, it is critical to remember that those emotions may be due to misunderstanding the other's verbal or nonverbal behavior and intentions.

In addition to increasing awareness, one can make behavioral changes as well. If time allows, doing background research on the groups with whom one regularly interacts can help one better understand their goals and needs. If one serves a group of people who speak a different language, learning a few phrases in that language will help them feel more comfortable. Careful observation of others' behavior and not assuming one knows the intentions behind it are also key. Although in some cultures beliefs and conventions may not always allow for complete forthrightness, learning active listening techniques can help one understand others better and can break down negative emotional barriers. In this way, one can create relationships and build trust, especially possible in longer term student-educator and professional-professional relationships, and in RN-patient relationships. Adapted from the scholarship of Carl Rogers,[56] such active listening techniques include the following:

1. In order to signify understanding and encourage further talk, one can acknowledge comprehension by providing back-channel behavior ("m-hm," "I see," nodding one's head as appropriate) and by repeating what the other says.
2. To seek clarification, interpret, check understanding, and test perceptions, one can do several speech acts: ask what the other means ("What does X mean?"), ask if the other can say more about the situation ("Can you tell me more about it?"), and request an example or experience ("Can you tell me about something that happened to make you think that?" or "Can you give me an example?").

3. To confirm understanding, one should clarify the interpretations of the other by again paraphrasing ("When you say X, you also mean Y, don't you?") and summarizing ("Let me see if I've understood you correctly. You said that . . .").[57]

When training with avatar patients or in actual RN-patient relationships the following policies also apply:

1. Be aware that cultural differences may exist, even if the patients are proficient in English.
2. Do not interrupt your patients as they try to explain their symptoms. Give them time to think and find the right words.
3. Ask open-ended questions. Patients may not provide all of the necessary information when asked yes or no questions.
4. After taking symptoms, ask the patients what they think caused the disease. This can give you insight into how best to explain the diagnosis.
5. To ensure patient comprehension, ask the patients to restate the treatment regimen. Do not depend solely on the pharmacist to provide information about medications.[58]

Seeking further understanding can be accomplished if one actually comes to know people better. In getting to know those who are from different backgrounds, one can develop trust and build relationships. If one's patient population is generally from a specific group, having relationships with similar people can open doors to learning more and to asking questions like the following: If you were preparing for an operation, what would bring comfort to you in the OR? Would touching you on the arm or on the forehead be a gesture of comfort? Would eye contact be valued or not? Would a soft tone of voice be soothing, even if a patient does not understand the words? In what other ways might a patient feel comforted, if I do not speak his or her language, and there is no interpreter present? Ultimately, however, patients value nurses' skills in caring for them.[59] Therefore, doing everything one can in one's professional role, given the constraints of the OR, will also be of comfort to many patients.

SUMMARY

To help humankind is perioperative nursing's raison d'être, and that help takes place on a number of levels: the physical, the emotional, the spiritual, and the interactive. With patients and health care professionals from very different backgrounds, it is in the interactive sphere where one can have a positive impact on the way in which the patient is able to accept care. Understanding and working with other people does not happen overnight. Once one learns that another's behavior is not due to a personality flaw, but rather to cross-cultural differences, one will find it easier to come to terms with the behavior, whether one agrees with it or not. The ideal is for both parties to understand these differences. As intercultural communication is better understood and practiced, the health of the patient is better served.

In a parallel fashion, access to further education and development, lifelong learning, is also critical in an ever-changing world. The cyber world does not replace the face-to-face world; it, however, adds quality. The cyber world affords the opportunity for more ways professionals engage in teaching and learning, for collaboration and dissemination of vital information, in order to effect better care and a better working environment. As technology becomes more accessible, usable, and cost-effective, there will be even more access, even more "haves."

So the haves online or off are those perioperative nursing professionals who are skilled in many ways, who seek continuing development, and are always cognizant of the key questions and answers that inform their lives: "Why are we here?" "Why did we get into this profession?" "What is our goal for our patients in the short- and long-term?" The answer is to help patients have physical, mental, emotional, and spiritual health and to work in an environment where people believe the right thing is happening. Successful cross-cultural communication is the glue that makes communication happen. Such a skill set should not stay in the OR, for successfully interacting with other human beings is a skill set for life beyond the world of the hospital, and for communication in a venue as close as one's private sphere, the home. We are all different from one another, to a degree, even those we love most dearly.

REFERENCES

1. US Department of Commerce: National Telecommunications and Information Administration. Digital nation: expanding Internet usage. February, 2011. Available at: http://www.ntia.doc.gov/report/2011/digital-nation-expanding-internet-usage-ntia-research-preview. Accessed January 17, 2012.
2. Martin S. FCC approves rural broadband push. USA Today. October 27, 2011. Available at: http://www.usatoday.com/tech/news/story/2011-10-27/fcc-rural-broadband-fund/50960016/1. Accessed January 17, 2012.
3. UPI.com. US funds broadband in rural areas. August 23, 2011. Available at: http://www.upi.com/Science_News/2011/08/23/US-funds-broadband-in-rural-areas/UPI-46221314137553/. Accessed January 17, 2012.
4. Venkatesh V. Determinants of perceived ease of use: integrating control, intrinsic motivation, and emotion into the technology. Information Systems Research 2000; 11(4):342–65.
5. Dresner E, Herring SC. Functions of the nonverbal in CMC: emoticons and illocutionary force. Communication Theory 2010;20:249–68.
6. Ess C, Sudweeks F. Culture and computer-mediated communication: toward new understandings. Journal of Computer-Mediated Communication 2006;11:179–91.
7. Cho B, Kwon U, Gentry JW, et al. Cultural values reflected in theme and execution: a comparative study of U.S. and Korean television commercials. Journal of Advertising 1999;28(4):59–73.
8. Seymour NE, Bansal VK. Virtual reality training improves operating room performance: results of a randomized, double-blinded study. Ann Surg 2002;236(4):458–64.
9. Witmer BG, Bailey JH, Knerr BW. Virtual spaces and real world places: transfer of route knowledge. International Journal of Human-Computer Studies 1996;45: 413–28.
10. Skiba DF. Nursing education 2.0: a second look at Second Life. Nurs Educ Perspect 2009;30(2):129–31.
11. Smart Hospital™. The University of Texas at Arlington. Available at: http://www.uta.edu/nursing/smarthospital. Accessed February 10, 2012.
12. Kolb DA. Experiential learning: experience as the source of learning and development. Englewood Cliffs (NJ): Prentice Hall; 1984.
13. Scollon R, Scollon SW. Nexus analysis: discourse and the emerging Internet. London: Routledge; 2004.
14. Fischer K. The Dallas ISD melting pot. Dallas Morning News. April 22, 2008. Available at: http://dallasisdblog.dallasnews.com/archives/2008/04/the-dallas-isd-melting-pot.html. Accessed February 1, 2012.
15. US Census Bureau. State and county quickfacts. Available at: http://quickfacts.census.gov/qfd/states/41/4159000.html. Accessed January 31, 2012.
16. Donnelly PL. Ethics and cross-cultural nursing. J Transcult Nurs 2000;11(2):119–26.

17. Nowak KL, Rauh C. The influence of the avatar on online perceptions of anthropomorphism, androgyny, credibility, homophily, and attraction. Journal of Computer-Mediated Communication 2005;11(1);8. Available at: http://jcmc.indiana.edu/vol11/issue1/nowak.html. Accessed February 13, 2012.

18. Colburn RA, Cohen MF, Drucker SM. The role of eye gaze in avatar mediated conversational interfaces [technical report MSR-TR-2000-81]. Redmond (WA): Microsoft Corporation; 2000.

19. Skiba DJ. Nursing education 2.0: second life. Nurs Educ Perspect 2007;28(3). Available at: http://www.freepatentsonline.com/article/Nursing-Education-Perspectives/164947756.html. Accessed January 25, 2012.

20. Campinha-Bacote J. The challenge of cultural diversity for nurse educators. J Contin Educ Nurs 1996;27(2):59–64.

21. Banks JA, Banks, CA, editors. Multicultural education: issues and perspectives. 7th edition. Hoboken (NJ): Wiley & Sons; 2010.

22. Hofstede G, Hofstede GJ, Minkov M. Cultures and organizations: software of the mind. 3rd edition. New York: McGraw-Hill; 2010.

23. Napholz L. A comparison of self-reported cultural competency skills among two groups of nursing students: implications for nursing education. J Nurs 1999;38(2): 81–3.

24. Betancourt, JR. Cross-cultural medical education: conceptual approaches and frameworks for evaluation. Acad Med 2003;78(6):560–9.

25. Campinha-Bacote J. Cultural competence in the delivery of healthcare services: a model of care. J Transcult Nurs 2002;13(3):181–4.

26. Gibbons LJ. Law and the emotive avatar. Vanderbilt Journal of Entertainment and Technology Law 2009;11(4):899–920.

27. Meta-Motion. Motion capture recording vs. realtime. Available at: http://www.metamotion.com/motion-capture/motion-capture-recording-vs-real-time.htm. Accessed February 1, 2012.

28. Hall ET. Proxemics. Current Anthropology 1968;9:83–108.

29. Hall ET. The hidden dimension. Garden City (NY): Doubleday; 1966.

30. Rings L. Cultural meaning in German verbal and nonverbal behavior and the teaching of German: a progress report. Unterrichtspraxis 1992;25(1):15–21.

31. Earley PC. Intercultural training for managers: a comparison of documentary and interpersonal methods. The Academy of Management Journal 1987;30(4):685–98.

32. Sadri HA, Flammia M. Intercultural communication: a new approach to international relations and global challenges. London: The Continuum International Publishing Group; 2011.

33. Garau M, Slater M, Bee S, et al. The impact of eye gaze on communication using humanoid avatars. SIGCHI'01 2001;3(1):309–16.

34. Henley NM. Status and sex: some touching observations. Bulletin of the Psychonomic Society 1973;2:91–3.

35. Hayakawa H. Laughter in Japanese communication [PhD dissertation]. University of Sydney (Australia); 2003.

36. Wierzbicka A. Semantics, culture, and cognition: universal human concepts in culture-specific configurations. New York: Oxford UP; 1992.

37. Wierzbicka A. English: meaning and culture. New York: Oxford UP; 2006.

38. Rosenberg CE, Golden J. Framing disease: studies in cultural history. Newark (NJ): Rutgers UP; 1992.

39. Austin JL. How to do things with words: the William James lectures. Oxford (England): Clarendon; 1962.

40. Rings L. [Beyond grammar and vocabulary: German and American differences in routine formulae and small talk]. Unterrichtspraxis 1994;27(2):23–8.
41. Scollon R, Scollon SW. Intercultural communication: a discourse approach. Cambridge (MA): Blackwell; 2001.
42. Byrnes H. Interactional style in German and American conversations. Text 1986;6(2): 189–206.
43. Watts RJ. Relevance and relational work: linguistic politeness as politic behavior. Multilingua 1989;8:131–66.
44. Wieland M. Turn-taking structure as a source of misunderstanding in French-American cross-cultural conversation. Pragmatics and Language Learning Monograph Series 1991;2:101–18.
45. Tannen D. When is an overlap not an interruption? One component of conversational style. In: Di Pietro RJ, Frawley W, Wedel A, editors. The first Delaware symposium on language studies. East Brunswick (NJ): Associated University Presses; 1983. p. 119–29.
46. Schank R, Abelson R. Scripts, plans, goals, and understanding: an inquiry into human knowledge structure. Hillsdale (NJ): Lawrence Erlbaum; 1977.
47. Marzorati G. Salman Rushdie: fiction's embattled infidel. The New York Times. January 29, 1989. Available at: http://www.nytimes.com/1989/01/29/magazine/salman-rushdie-fiction-s-embattled-infidel.html. Accessed January 18, 2012.
48. Hojat M, Nasca TJ, Cohen, MJ, et al. Attitudes toward physician-nurse collaboration: a cross-cultural study of male and female physicians and nurses in the United States and Mexico. Nurs Res 2001;50(2):123–8.
49. Lingard L, Reznick R, Espin S, et al. Team communications in the operating room: talk patterns, sites of tension, and implications for novices. Acad Med 2002;77:232–7.
50. Schroeder R. Social interaction in virtual environments: key issues, common themes, and a framework for research. In: Schroeder R, editor. The social life of avatars: presence and interaction in shared virtual environments. London: Springer-Verlag Limited; 2002. p. 1–18.
51. Lastowka G. User-generated content and virtual worlds. Vanderbilt Journal of Entertainment and Technology Law 2008;10(4):893–917.
52. Boulos MN, Hetherington L, Wheeler S. Second life: an overview of the potential of 3-D virtual worlds in medical and health education. Health Info Libr J 2007;24:233–45.
53. Thompson LA, Dawson K, Ferdig R, et al. The intersection of online social networking with medical professionalism. J Gen Intern Med 2008;23(7):954–7.
54. Barnes SB. A privacy paradox: social networking in the United States. First Monday 2006;11(9):11–5.
55. Cain J. Online social networking issues within academia and pharmacy education. Am J Pharm Educ 2008;72(1):10.
56. Rogers C. Client-centered psychotherapy. Boston: Houghton-Mifflin; 1951.
57. Rings L. The oral interview and cross-cultural understanding in the foreign language classroom. Foreign Language Annals 2006;39(1):43–53.
58. May SE. "Does your throat hurt more in the morning or throughout the day?" "Yes.": intercultural medical discourse [PhD dissertation]. Arlington (TX): University of Texas at Arlington; 2007. Available at: http://hdl.handle.net/10106/764. Accessed January 27, 2012.
59. Greenslade JH, Jimmieson NL. Organizational factors impacting on patient satisfaction: a cross sectional examination of service climate and linkages to nurses' effort and performance. Int J Nurs Stud 2011;48(10):1188–98.

Getting Caught in the Legal Net of Social Networking

Nancy Roper Willson, RN, JD, MSN, MA

KEYWORDS

- Nursing boundaries • Social networking • License discipline

KEY POINTS

- Inappropriate use of social networking sites can have legal consequences for the nurse.
- A common complaint against the nurse for social networking misuse is failure to maintain professional boundaries.
- When a nurse is fatigued and overwhelmed, the nurse is particularly vulnerable for misuse of social networking sites.

To some nurses of a certain age and/or aptitude, terms such as Twitter, blog, and Facebook are part of their native tongue. For others, these terms are part of a foreign language that they struggle to comprehend. However, no matter how familiar or foreign the Internet and social networking sites are for nurses, many are making bad professional judgment calls that are leading to termination from employment, discipline by their licensing boards, and even embarrassment in the witness seats at trials.

There are several common legal complaints that may be made against a nurse who uses social networking sites in an inappropriate manner. These include defamation, violation of the Health Insurance Portability and Accountability Act (HIPAA), and violation of a state's nursing practice act or a licensing board's rules or regulations. Whereas many employers now have policies and procedures to guide their nurse employees as to what the employer considers acceptable use of social networking and the Internet in the workplace, these policies can vary widely as to what is viewed as appropriate. In one facility, a nurse-employee may be instructed that while at work he/she may not have any access to his/her personal smartphone, at another facility the proscription may only involve not using personal phones while at the patient's bedside or in the patient's room. Similarly, Internet access may be very restricted for employees in one facility and virtually without restriction at another facility.

The author has nothing to disclose.
College of Nursing, University of Texas at Arlington, 411 South Nedderman Drive, Box 19407, Arlington, TX 76019-0407, USA
E-mail address: willson@uta.edu

Perioperative Nursing Clinics 7 (2012) 283–286
doi:10.1016/j.cpen.2012.03.001
1556-7931/12/$ – see front matter © 2012 Published by Elsevier Inc.
periopnursing.theclinics.com

Even with policies and procedures in place, for some the temptation is too great not to engage in personal social networking while at work. Often, this happens when a nurse has had a particularly difficult and stressful shift and the need to vent to "friends" is indulged. Of course, not only does inappropriate venting occur when the nurse is at work but also after the nurse has left the workplace. Also, often the nurse is lulled into a false sense that he/she is "not doing anything wrong" because the patient's name, room number, or some other type of identifier is not used or because the posting on the social network is restricted to a select group of friends and is therefore private. A lack of knowledge of HIPAA or understanding of how social networking sites save and disseminate information may be involved. But often the basic lack of knowledge is a thorough understanding of the professionalism component of appropriately using social networking. This professionalism component includes the concept of maintaining professional boundaries.

Though I have been a defense attorney who has represented nurses before the state licensing board for over 20 years for a multitude of allegations, it has been only in the last couple of years that I have begun to have clients who were under licensing investigations due to their social networking postings. It is a growing area of risk for nurses and other professionals. A licensing board's approach to perceived inappropriate social networking often is based on the allegation that the nurse has failed to maintain the professional nurse-patient boundary. A nurse may just as easily cross the nurse-patient boundary on a social networking site as in a face-to-face encounter with the patient. Whether in-person or on the Internet, the nurse is the part of the nurse-patient dyad who is responsible for setting and maintaining professional boundaries. In the section under professional boundaries, the American Nurses Association's (ANA) code of ethics states, "When acting within one's role as a professional, the nurse recognizes and maintains boundaries that establish appropriate limits to relationships."[1] Therefore, maintaining professional boundaries is an element of safe patient care and the expectation that the nurse will maintain the patient's dignity through protection of confidential information to which the nurse becomes privy in the course of his/her provision of care to the patient. Perhaps the clearest way to understand boundaries and how strictly they are being interpreted is to always ask the question, "Do I have a dual relationship with this patient?" Dual relationships are to be avoided if at all possible. Are you attempting to be the patient's professional caregiver as well as their Facebook friend? Are you the patient's caregiver as well as the person who is serving up confidential details about him/her for your stress relief as well as for your friend's amusement?

The following scenarios are based on, though not identical to, actual recent cases in which the nurse involved was either under investigation for misconduct by her/his employer, under investigation for crossing professional boundaries by the state nursing board, or subject to actual public licensing disciplinary action by the state nursing board. The first two scenarios are examples of incidents that did not lead to disciplinary action by the board, but employment consequences occurred. The third scenario did involve a licensing disciplinary action.

SCENARIO 1: ACCESSING A SOCIAL NETWORKING SITE WHILE AT WORK

Nurse A was having a particularly stressful week at work. This was her third, consecutive 12-hour shift in a week in which each shift had proved to be unusually busy with routine and surprising events. Nurse A later said that she was feeling overwhelmed by everything that had been going on over the past couple of days. An incident occurred in which one of Nurse A's elderly patients attempted to harm himself in his hospital room. While waiting for transport to take the patient to a more secure psychiatric unit, Nurse A went on her Facebook site and posted that one of her patient's had just attempted suicide and described the method by which the attempt was made. Nurse A stated the age of the patient but did not name the patient, nor did she state the patient's room number. However, on her Facebook site she did have personal information including that she was a registered nurse (RN), and on what unit and in which hospital she was employed. Two of her friends responded with comforting comments to her, but both asked for more information, which she did not give.

On Nurse A's Facebook site were other nurses who also worked on her unit. One of these friend-colleagues, who was not working that shift, saw the posting and called the unit manager, who also was not on the unit at the time, to find out more details as to the incident. This was the first notification that the unit manager had that there had been a problem on the unit and she understandably was not happy to be hearing about unit emergencies from an employee who got the information from a social networking site. At the time she made the posting, Nurse A did stop and consider HIPAA implications but did not feel that it was a violation. She quickly grasped that even if an action does not rise to the level of a HIPAA violation, misconduct and failure to maintain professional boundaries may still be very much in consideration.

SCENARIO 2: ACCESSING A SOCIAL NETWORKING SITE WHILE IN THE PERIOPERATIVE DEPARTMENT

Nurse B worked in a small town in which most residents knew one another. Nurse B also was tired and stressed from a hectic night in the operating room. Things had just begun to settle down a bit when Nurse B got a call that the paramedics were on the way with a man who nearly had severed his leg with a chain saw while attempting to cut down a tree in his yard. Nurse B accessed his social networking site and posted, "Just when you think it can't get any better, you get a call that EMTs [emergency medical technicians] are in route with a yahoo who almost cut off his own leg playing with a chainsaw."

Again, fellow nurses with whom Nurse B worked saw the posting and brought it to the manager's attention. However, in this situation, Nurse B's posting was to a site on which he did not have his place of employment, the town in which he worked, or even the exact same name by which people knew him. Even though the incident did not lead to a licensing disciplinary action, Nurse B was investigated for failure to maintain professional boundaries. Nurse B certainly took the incident seriously and made no further postings involving patients on his site.

SCENARIO 3: ACCESSING A SOCIAL NETWORKING SITE WHILE CARING FOR DEMANDING PATIENTS

Nurse C worked on a general medical-surgical floor. She also was feeling stressed and overwhelmed by the demands that had been made on her most of the night by 3 very time-intensive patients. While still at work, she began to blog back and forth with a very good friend of hers. She began to state in very explicit language what she would like to do to her patients. With every post her friend would respond with requests for more information. Then Nurse C began to post as if she actually had done certain things to the patients, such as severely overmedicating them to get them to leave her alone for a while.

Someone read the postings, found them highly offensive, and made a complaint against Nurse C, leading to an investigation and subsequent disciplinary action by the licensing board. Nurse C later stated that she would never actually harm a patient and that she had just been engaging in fantasy and one-upmanship with her friend with whom she was posting her comments. The licensing board, however, believed that Nurse C had crossed professional boundaries. Her license was placed under disciplinary action for 1 year, which required certain clinical restrictions, educational courses, and periodic reports to the licensing board by her employer. Additionally, the board required her to be evaluated by a licensed psychologist due to some of the extreme comments she made about the patients.

Though the settings and actions of the nurses in the 3 scenarios differed, the commonality was that the nurses were all frustrated, stressed, tired, and feeling overwhelmed and they used social networking in order to ventilate their feelings. The purpose of this article is not to argue the fine nuances of HIPAA and other potential legal theories but rather to emphasize that what may seem like innocuous venting of feelings to the nurse may in effect be perceived by others as a violation of a nurse's duty to the patient and a failure to conduct oneself in an expected professional manner. In other words, employment and licensing consequences may result due to the broad wording of an employer's policy or a state's practice act or a licensing board's rule.

Two useful guides are published by the National Council of State Boards of Nursing and can be accessed and downloaded from their website.

1. "A Nurse's Guide to the Use of Social Media." This guide provides the nurse with helpful information and explanatory scenarios in both written and video formats. It also suggests the ways by which the nurse can avoid disclosing confidential information about the patient.[2]
2. "A Nurse's Guide to Professional Boundaries." This guide provides the nurse with helpful information and examples to assist in understanding professional nurse-patient boundaries.[3]

SUMMARY

Legal requirements and expectations for a professional who engages in social networking is a rapidly developing area of law. Aspects of social networking, including what an employee may have a free-speech right to post as an individual when not in the employee role, is just one topic that attorneys, judges, and legislators are debating for professionals. Many articles are being published that are educating and providing guidance to professionals from various disciplines, including nursing. Whether adept with the medium of social networking or amateurish, some nurses are exercising poor judgment when it comes to patients and social networking postings. This poor judgment often goes along with frustration and fatigue. The consequences of poor judgment can lead to problems in the employment and licensing realms. The nurse needs to be familiar with and adhere to the employer's policy regarding use of the Internet, personal phones, and social networking, as well as knowledgeable about the licensing board's laws and rules that apply to social networking.

REFERENCES

1. American Nurses Association. Code of ethics for nurses with interpretive statements. Silver Spring (MD): American Nurses Association; 2001.
2. National Council of State Boards of Nursing. A nurse's guide to the use of social media. Available at: https://www.ncsbn.org/3487.htm. Accessed March 7, 2012.
3. National Council of State Boards of Nursing. A nurse's guide to professional boundaries. Available at: https://www.ncsbn.org/2551.htm. Accessed March 7, 2012.

Index

Note: Page numbers of article titles are in **boldface** type.

A

Access database program, 212, 219–220
Accessibility, of information, 157–159
Accuracy, of information, 192–193
Active listening, 278–279
A.D.A.M. graphics, 204
Administration, informatics for, 155, 174–175
Adobe ConnectPro, 164
Adult learning theory, 252
Advance Practice Nurse degree, 172
Allen e-mail sorting categories, 229
American Nurses Association, nursing informatics definition of, 151–153
Amount used, of copyrighted material, 207
Assessment tools, for evaluating information, 191–193
Association of periOperative Registered Nurses (AORN, Inc.), data sets of, 155
Asynchronous online courses, 164–167
Authenticity, of information, 192–193
Authority, of information, 190–193
Autobiographical memory, in Personal Information Management, 227
Avatars, in virtual world environment, 238–240, 246, 269–279
Awareness, of cultural differences, 278–279

B

Barreau e-mail filing systems, 229
Behavior, cultural differences in, 278–279
Bibliographic management software, **195–200**
   EndNote, 196–197, 213
   Refworks, 197–199, 213
Bing search engine, 183
Biological Abstracts database, 184–185
Blended classes, 163
Blogs, 166–167
Books, web sites for, 183–184
Boolean operators, 183
Boundaries, in general systems theory, 153

C

Calculations, in spreadsheets, 214–215
Camtasia, in webcasts, 167
Captivate, in webcasts, 167

http://dx.doi.org/10.1016/S1556-7931(12)00042-3
1556-7931/12/$ – see front matter © 2012 Elsevier Inc. All rights reserved.
periopnursing.theclinics.com

Moving?

Make sure your subscription moves with you!

To notify us of your new address, find your **Clinics Account Number** (located on your mailing label above your name), and contact customer service at:

Email: journalscustomerservice-usa@elsevier.com

800-654-2452 (subscribers in the U.S. & Canada)
314-447-8871 (subscribers outside of the U.S. & Canada)

Fax number: 314-447-8029

Elsevier Health Sciences Division
Subscription Customer Service
3251 Riverport Lane
Maryland Heights, MO 63043

*To ensure uninterrupted delivery of your subscription,
please notify us at least 4 weeks in advance of move.

Printed and bound by CPI Group (UK) Ltd, Croydon, CR0 4YY

03/10/2024

01040446-0013